Cracking the Egg Myth

PROVEN WAYS TO IMPROVE EGG QUALITY

Julie Chang, L.Ac.

Cracking the Egg Myth/ Julie Chang, L.Ac. 1st ed

ISBN: 978-1658797535

Table of Contents

To all women... the power of creation is within you. Believe in yourself to allow it to manifest your heart's desires.

Introduction

Although this book applies to anyone trying to get pregnant, it is meant for women who are typically given very few choices.

This book is for you if:

- You are over 35 years of age, perhaps in your 40s.

- You have been diagnosed with low AMH, high FSH, premature ovarian failure (POF), premature ovarian insufficiency (POI), poor egg quality, diminished ovarian reserve (DOR), or advanced maternal age (AMA).

- You've been told by your fertility doctors that it's too late for you to get pregnant with your own eggs so you should consider donor eggs.

Whether you're trying to get pregnant the good old-fashioned way or with the help of your fertility doctor, this book will help you improve your fertility naturally.

Many of you don't know what to do because you're stuck on how to move forward. For you, let this book be your light to keep your dream alive.

The stories in the following pages are of actual clients I have helped overcome what seemed like insurmountable odds. All names have been changed to protect their privacy. But they are very real people. Women from all parts of the world with different sizes and shapes, income levels, relationship statuses, and sexual orientations. For ease, fictional names common in the U.S. are used since names from different cultures may be more identifiable.

Draw strength and hope from their stories as you figure out your journey.

You are not alone!

Many others share your story and have beaten the odds to have their own biological child.

Although this book was written with recommendations distilled from published studies, getting pregnant is more than the mechanics of what your ovaries and uterus do. Your ability to get pregnant is neither limited to the numbers on your blood test results nor any label your doctor gives you.

You are a beautifully complex woman. In order to be more successful on your fertility journey, honor your body in its entirety – mind, body, and spirit.

Look at fertility from a holistic viewpoint - your reproductive system is connected to the rest of your body. That means eating nutrient-dense foods, taking the right supplements, exercising, reducing stress, and giving your emotional health the same importance as your physical health. These components are ALL important to giving yourself the best chance of success.

To that end, many recommendations are provided in this book. There may be more information than you know what to do with. That's okay because every person reading this book is at a different stage on their path.

Your job is to sift through the information and implement what makes sense to you, given your level of interest, time, money, and energy. You don't have to do everything.

Just do what makes you feel better.

Your emotions are your GPS—they will guide you to the right action. You're looking for inspired action springing from a sense of well-being rather than actions born out of desperation or for the sake of checking something off your list.

It's better to do less with ease than more with dread or resentment. You don't need to be Superwoman.

Most importantly, create a lifestyle you enjoy so that your fertility journey is filled with happy moments and opportunities for expansion and, most important of all, creation.

Life is mostly filled with the in-between moments on your way to your desires. So enjoy the ride!

CHAPTER 1

Why is Getting Pregnant More Difficult Now

Amy's Story

After two unsuccessful years of trying to get pregnant naturally, followed by three rounds of insemination, and finally two cycles of in vitro fertilization (IVF), Amy thought that she had exhausted all her options to conceive.

At 42 years old, she felt hopeless because time was running out. As a last ditch effort, she came to me to see if she could do more to improve her chances using her own eggs. She figured she had nothing to lose at that point.

Since she was still having regular menstrual cycles, getting pregnant naturally was still possible. But I advised her that unless she was willing to make drastic lifestyle changes, her chances would not improve significantly.

Highly stressed from working long hours, she often ate out with her coworkers for lunch and ordered takeout for dinner to eat in front of the TV with her husband. Her ovulation predictor kit dictated their intimacy.

Overhauling her life to one where she worked less, ate better foods, practiced self-care, and nurtured her relationship with her spouse took over one year of commitment and focus. Her efforts were rewarded when she emailed me a picture of her pregnancy test. At age 43, she was finally pregnant and had a healthy baby.

Amy's story is similar to many of my clients. As time passes with no pregnancy, hope often fades until eventually a woman gives up trying. Although the chances of getting pregnant decrease as you get older, there are certainly measures to slow down the aging process or reverse it to some degree, as Amy experienced.

As you age, your cells become less efficient. Like a car, the parts wear down over time and with use.

Part of the reason for the decreased efficiency is that the longer you're alive on this planet, the more toxins you're exposed to. Those toxins accumulate in your cells to impair all functions, including those that will help you get pregnant.

Your metabolism slows, so you have to watch what you're eating. You can't run as fast. Your vision worsens. Your skin is less youthful. You're more forgetful.

Your eggs are just as vulnerable as any other cells to the effects of aging.

This is why your chances of getting pregnant decrease as you get older. Any online fertility calculator will show your odds declining each year. The fertility statistics are dismal as you get further into your forties.

In fact, pregnancy chances get so low that fertility specialists known as reproductive endocrinologists (REs) either recommend doing in vitro fertilization (IVF) right away or going straight to donor eggs.

But don't worry, you may still be able to conceive. Naturally or with IVF.

Before we get to the good news, let's understand a little more of the medical side of fertility treatments. We will look at the options for fertility and then go into what the fertility doctors test for and what the results may mean.

What are your options for fertility?

A fertility doctor can explain your options for IVF or other assistive reproductive technology (ART) methods, such as hormonal stimulation.

- **Insemination:** Often, insemination is the first assisted medical procedure a woman does when trying naturally has been unsuccessful. It involves the doctor placing the sperm in the uterus.

- **In Vitro Fertilization:** For many women, IVF is offered as the best option for getting pregnant. But it isn't for everyone. Financially, it may not be covered very well by your health insurance. Unfortunately, this makes money a limiting factor for many couples. The success rate of IVF varies by fertility clinic. Recent data shows that the birth rate from IVF ranges from 3% to 35% for women over age 35. [1]

- **Donor eggs for IVF:** If your doctor determines you no longer have viable egg cells, using an egg donor will likely be the recommended route.

- **Surrogacy:** For some families, using a gestational surrogate mother to carry the baby may be the best avenue.

- **Adoption:** This is a wonderful option for many families!

- **Embryo adoption:** A lesser known alternative, adopting a frozen embryo from another couple allows a woman to experience pregnancy and the early stages of a newborn baby.

- **Natural fertility solutions:** Many women turn to natural solutions when assisted reproductive techniques aren't a good option, not their first choice, or want to do whatever they can to optimize their success.

And natural fertility solutions are what this book is all about!

The rest of this guide will dive into the science of your reproductive system and explain research-backed natural solutions for enhancing fertility.

While the focus here is on natural fertility, you can still pursue other options, such as insemination, IVF, donor eggs, surrogacy, or embryo adoption. In fact, improving your fertility naturally will increase your chances of success regardless of which method you use.

CHAPTER 2

Fertility Specialists and Testing: Making Sense of the Details

How do fertility doctors determine if you can still get pregnant? With blood tests and ultrasounds.

You may come out of the process feeling a bit like a pin cushion or a lab specimen. But your fertility doctor should thoroughly test to see if there is a physical cause for your infertility.

Abdominal and transvaginal ultrasounds are a way that your doctor can get a glimpse of what is going on inside. They can rule out physical problems, such as scar tissue, blocked fallopian tubes, and abnormalities in the ovaries or uterus.

Blood tests will determine your reproductive hormone levels. Usually a standard wellness panel is also run to make sure that nothing abnormal is going on.

If there aren't physical abnormalities, the fertility doctor will usually check your antral follicle count (defined below) to get an idea of how many follicle cells you have. Your anti-Müllerian hormones (defined below) will be measured as another way of testing your ovarian reserve. If you have stopped menstruating early, you will be evaluated for premature ovarian failure.

Let's get into the details on what all of these tests mean.

What is an antral follicle count ultrasound?

The antral follicle count ultrasound is a tool used by many fertility doctors often on your first visit. The ultrasound visualizes how many potential eggs you may have—the basal antral follicle count (AFC). Antral follicles are cells that are big enough to see with an ultrasound.

The AFC can give an indication of your ovarian reserve or how many eggs you have left.

An antral (resting) follicle is a small, fluid-filled sac that contains an immature egg. Follicles are not the same thing as eggs. However, they're often used interchangeably, even by the medical profession, creating a lot of confusion. What you see with the baseline AFC ultrasound are not your eggs, but the follicles that your eggs are in. You need a microscope to see an egg. It's too small to see with an ultrasound.

Development of an egg cell

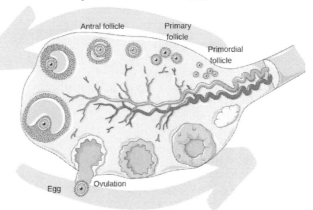

The antral follicles are a good predictor of the number of mature follicles in a woman's ovaries that can be stimulated by IVF medications. The number of eggs retrieved from those follicles correlates directly with IVF success rates. The more eggs retrieved, the better the results expected from the IVF.

Remember that bag of goldfish you got from the state fair when you were a girl? Think of the bag as the follicle, the water as the follicular fluid, and the egg as the goldfish. Remember that image whenever you hear follicle.

Expanding on that image, your goldfish needs a lot to survive: a bag that is big enough to hold it, enough water, and the nutrients it needs to grow.

AMH (anti-Müllerian hormone) Test: What does it mean?

One of the first tests a fertility doctor does is to check the anti-Müllerian hormone (AMH) level in your blood. Finding out that you have low AMH levels can be a devastating experience, leading to feeling despair in your quest to get pregnant. But all hope is not lost. It is still possible to get pregnant with a low AMH.

Are your chances of getting pregnant decreased due to low AMH levels or low ovarian reserve? Yes.

Does low AMH or low AFC mean that you can't get pregnant? Absolutely not!

Yes, you're born with all the eggs you will have. Unlike men who constantly make sperm, you can't make more eggs.

What can you do to improve your chances of getting pregnant naturally or with IVF? A lot!

What is AMH, and when is it checked?

On the third day of your menstrual cycle, doctors look at your blood hormone levels to gauge your fertility potential.

One of the most important fertility hormones tested is your AMH level. Anti-Müllerian hormone (AMH) is a hormone secreted by the follicles in your ovaries. It is a way for doctors to estimate ovarian reserve and your chances for pregnancy with in-vitro fertilization (IVF).

When they are beginning to mature, those follicles secrete anti-Müllerian hormone. The amount of AMH correlates to your ovarian reserve or the number of follicle cells you have. Thus, AMH levels are highest after puberty, and levels fall over the course of your reproductive years. When you reach menopause, the levels of AMH are nearly undetectable.

Each follicle is a fluid-filled sac that contains one immature egg. During ovulation, the follicle releases a mature egg.

What is a normal AMH level?

Below is a chart showing normal AMH levels for adult women prior to menopause.

AMH Blood Level	Interpretation
Over 3.0 ng/ml	High (indicator of PCOS)
Over 1.0 ng/ml	Normal
0.7 - 0.9 ng/ml	Below Normal
0.3 - 0.6 ng/ml	Low
Less than 0.3 ng/ml	Very Low

But wait, what is a normal AMH level for your age?

AMH levels decline as you get older, so you may be wondering if your lower AMH is where it should be for your age.

A recent study found that for women who do not have polycystic ovarian syndrome (PCOS), the average AMH levels were:

Age	AMH Level
Ages 20-31	2.35 ng/mL
Ages 32-34	1.58 ng/mL
Ages 35-37	1.30 ng/mL
Ages 38-43	0.96 - 1.05 ng/mL
Over 43	0.67 ng/mL

The study also found that women with PCOS have abnormally high AMH levels.[1] This is due to each of the small follicles producing more AMH than normal, thus driving the higher levels.

Low AMH only correlates with fertility in women who are over age 30. Low AMH levels in healthy women in their mid-20s do not predict reduced ability to get pregnant.[2]

Megan's Story

With tears in her eyes, Megan told me her AMH level was very low at 0.10 ng/ml. She was heartbroken when during their initial consultation, her doctor emphatically told her she couldn't get pregnant with her own eggs, so she would need to use donor eggs.

At 38 years old, she wasn't expecting to hear this and thought she had more time. Shocked at such an extreme recommendation without trying any other treatments first, Megan did her own research online to see what other options she had. She found me and implemented everything I recommended.

She needed the most help in changing her nutrition. She was quite lean for her build, which indicated that she probably wasn't getting the right nutrition to promote pregnancy. As expected, her diet was primarily plant-based. Although she ate healthy food, she needed to decrease her carbs and add more healthy fats and protein. Like many women worried about eating too much fat and animal protein, especially red meat, she was avoiding foods that provided important nutrients for a pregnancy and overcompensating by eating too many healthy carbs, like oatmeal, quinoa, and beans. Over the nine months she worked with me, she gained a little weight and was able to get pregnant naturally.

Megan's story is not unusual. It shows that you can still get pregnant with low AMH. It is just statistically more difficult, and this is why fertility doctors often suggest IVF or an egg donor to increase the odds.

Can you still get pregnant with low AMH?

For women under age 35, the percentage who were able to get pregnant naturally with low or very low AMH levels ranged from 28 to 41%.[3]

Another study which included women aged 21 - 42 noted, "Natural conception was observed in women with a wide range of AMH levels, including women with undetectable serum-AMH."[4]

So yes, natural pregnancy is possible with low AMH levels.

For many women, an egg donor is not an option due to financial costs or the desire to have her own biological child. If that is you, read on to find out ways to help increase your odds of getting pregnant with low AMH.

How can you improve your AMH level?

If you are looking for natural, herbal-based solutions for low AMH, a few studies point to the efficacy of specific herbs in raising AMH levels.

Curcumin:

Animal studies show that curcumin can increase AMH levels and protect against premature ovarian failure.[5] Curcumin is the main therapeutic compound found in turmeric.

Turmeric, a plant of the ginger family, is commonly used as a spice in cooking. It can also be sliced and steeped in hot water for turmeric tea.

Traditional Chinese Medicine

Traditional Chinese medicine (TCM) has been used for thousands of years to help with all kinds of ailments, including problems with conceiving. Modern science is beginning to test and understand how these herbal combinations work.

- An animal study tested a specific Chinese herbal formula and found that it significantly improved AMH levels in an animal model of diminished ovarian reserve.[6]

- An overview of studies on Chinese herbal medicine found that it was both safe and effective for women dealing with infertility.[7]

- A case study of a woman with low AMH and a history of failed IVF showed that in her case a traditional Chinese herbal blend was effective in restoring ovulation.[8]

One of the herbs used in both formulas was *Angelica sinensis* or *dang gui*. This is an herb that has been used in TCM for thousands of years to help with women's reproductive

14

disorders. An overview that analyzed a number of studies and clinical trials on TCM for infertility showed that *Angelica sinensis* was a component of almost all of the formulas used.[9]

Unlike supplements or Western herbs, Chinese herbal medicine is usually prescribed as a formula with many ingredients. Because of the complexity of these formulas, working with a trained herbalist, often an acupuncturist with herbal training, is the best way to obtain the most benefit.

Are there dietary interventions for improving AMH?

The research on improving AMH is scant, but a handful of studies help to answer this question.

Keep in mind that you want higher AMH levels, within normal range, to increase your odds of pregnancy.

Although being overweight or obese may contribute to fertility issues for some women, drastic sudden weight loss is *not* recommended. In fact, losing weight very rapidly with bariatric surgery or restrictive dieting has been shown in studies to lower AMH.[10]

If you have low AMH levels, this is not the time to go on a crash diet. Instead, a whole food, minimally processed nutritional plan, including nutrient-dense proteins like eggs and wild fish, healthy fats, such as coconut oil and olive oil, and organic vegetables, may help optimize your body for conception and aid with gradual weight loss if needed.

A dietary analysis of almost 300 women, aged 35-45, found as polyunsaturated fat increased, especially omega-6, the women's AMH levels decreased.[11]

The link to high omega-6 intake and decreased AMH levels could be due to those women eating higher amounts of fried food. Corn, soybean, and sunflower oil are all high in omega-6 fatty acids. One more really good reason to skip the drive-thru line and avoid fried foods!

Getting enough nutrients is also important to AMH levels. Conditions that decrease the absorption of nutrients, such as celiac and Crohn's disease, are linked to lower AMH levels.[12][13]

What else can I do to increase my anti-Müllerian hormone levels?

Research shows us several toxins, if exposed to them on a daily basis, can decrease your AMH levels.

Several studies have linked higher levels of bisphenol A (BPA) to lower AMH levels.

- One study found that most of the women participants had BPA in their body and that those in the top half of BPA levels had about a 22% decrease in AMH.[14]

- Another study found that 100% of the participants had detectable BPA in their body. This study also linked increased BPA with decreased AMH.[15]

Avoiding BPA completely can be difficult, but even reducing your exposure level partially could make a difference. Common sources of BPA include:

- Eating foods and drinks, including most sodas, in metal cans with linings that contain BPA

- Eating foods packaged in plastics that contain BPA

- Absorbing BPA through skin contact with thermal printed cash register receipts

Pesticide exposure has also been linked with decreased AMH levels. A study of women in China found that higher levels of organochloride pesticides were associated with lower anti-Müllerian hormone.[16]

Another study involving women in rural South Africa found that exposure to pyrethroid pesticides was associated with a 25% decrease in AMH levels.[17]

Titanium dioxide nanoparticles, which can be found in sunscreens and other cosmetics, have been shown to decrease AMH levels in animal studies.[18]

Choosing organic vegetables and fruits and avoiding most packaged foods will help decrease your pesticide exposure.

Another lifestyle factor that you can control is staying active. In a study, moderate exercise increased AMH levels.[19]

6 science-backed steps that you can take today to raise low AMH levels:

o Eat whole, unprocessed, nutrient-dense foods, such as grass-fed meat, wild fish, pasture-raised eggs, organic vegetables, and healthy fats.

o Avoid fried foods and limit omega-6 oils, such as corn, soybean, and sunflower oils.

o Add in curcumin, either as a supplement or in your foods each day.

o Avoid BPA exposure as much as possible. Don't use plastic containers for warming foods. Check the labels to make sure your canned foods are BPA free. Avoid handling thermal printed receipts as much as possible.

o Stay away from pesticides, such as pyrethroids, which are found in many household insecticides. Choose organic fruits and produce as much as possible.

o Avoid sunscreen or cosmetics with titanium dioxide. Check product labels.

If you are dealing with low AMH levels, stack all of these action steps together. This is the time to go all in to clean up your diet, avoid pesticides and toxins, and add the right nutrients!

CHAPTER 3

A Diagnosis of Primary Ovarian Insufficiency

If you have stopped having your periods well before the normal age of menopause, one diagnosis that your fertility specialist may discuss with you is primary ovarian insufficiency.

The term primary ovarian insufficiency (POI) refers to when the ovaries stop working before the age of 40. It is also called premature ovarian failure (POF).

The average age for menopause is around 50, but there is a wide range of ages that is still considered normal. Women start going through normal menopause anywhere from age 42 to 54. The absence of menstruation before 40 with follicles still remaining is considered POI.

What causes primary ovarian insufficiency?

When the number of follicles in the ovaries drops below 1000, menstruation usually ceases. This is accompanied by ovarian hormonal changes, such as an increase in follicle stimulating hormone and a decrease in estradiol.

In most cases, one of three things causes POI:

- Genetics
- Chemotherapy, radiation, or surgery
- Autoimmune condition

POI (or POF) occurs in less than 1% of women.

Can you still get pregnant if you have primary ovarian insufficiency?

Yes! In POI, you have follicle cells still available. But these follicle cells have stopped progressing to the point of ovulation.

The odds of spontaneous pregnancy are low. About 5 to 10% of women with POI will end up getting pregnant without intervention.[1]

The key is what researchers refer to as activating dormant primordial follicles. Signaling between the cells needs to be activated to turn the dormant follicles into maturing follicles.

Several different cell signaling pathways can be targeted through diet and lifestyle changes.

Natural solutions for POI

mTOR activation

Mechanistic target of rapamycin, or mTOR, is a key protein in cell signaling. It is a signal determined by nutrients in the body that promotes cell growth. mTOR needs to balance at the right level and at the right time in the body. As people get older, decreasing mTOR helps to promote healthy longevity. However, when you are trying to get pregnant, you need more mTOR activity in the dormant follicle cells.

Activating mTOR in the dormant follicles has been shown in studies to cause the follicles to go ahead and mature, allowing for pregnancy.[2]

Simple, natural ways to activate mTOR without medications or negative side effects can be incorporated into your lifestyle.

Resistance exercise, such as moderate weight lifting has been shown to activate mTOR.[3]

Getting enough protein in your diet will activate mTOR. Or to put it another way, restricting protein decreases mTOR, so make sure you are eating a balanced diet that contains all the essential amino acids.[4]

It is also important to make sure that you are getting enough protein when you exercise. Studies show that protein in the form of branched-chain amino acids along with exercise is a way to activate mTOR.

Optimize your methylation cycle

One way that your body regulates which proteins and cellular molecules get produced is through methylation. The DNA in your cell nucleus is transcribed and translated by RNA into the proteins needed in your cells. This process goes on all the time in all of your cells. One way for your body to turn off genes that don't need to be transcribed is through methylation.

Methylation refers to adding a methyl group to something in your cells, whether it is added to a protein to change it into another protein or using that methyl group to turn off the transcription of a gene.

Turning off a signaling molecule in your ovaries can limit the activation of the primordial follicle cells.

You can do a lot through diet or supplements to optimize your methylation cycle. Case studies show that for some women this can help to restart ovulation in POI.[5]

Two main dietary factors influence your methylation cycle: folate and choline. Good sources of folate include liver, asparagus, broccoli, egg yolks, leafy greens, and lentils. Eggs and liver are also excellent sources of choline along with caviar, salmon, and beef.

Supplements to help your methylation cycle include adding methylfolate (not folic acid) and vitamins B12, B6, and B2.

Check your thyroid hormone levels

The link between hypothyroidism and POI isn't completely understood. However, several studies and case reports show that hypothyroidism can be a cause of POI.

Women with the autoimmune condition Hashimoto's thyroiditis are three times more likely to have POI.[6]

If you have been diagnosed with primary ovarian insufficiency, getting a thorough thyroid check is a good idea. Supporting your thyroid health with nourishing foods is essential for everyone.

Avoid cigarette smoke exposure

We all know that cigarette smoking isn't good for us for many reasons, including lowering your ability to get pregnant. Smoking is strongly linked to premature menopause and primary ovarian insufficiency. Studies estimate that smoking more than doubles your risk of infertility due to POI or premature menopause.[7]

If you are a smoker, now is the time to seek help and find a way to stop. If you are living with someone who smokes indoors, find ways to eliminate the indoor smoke and restore your living spaces to a smoke-free area.

Debbie's Story

For Debbie, acupuncture was her saving grace. She came to me at 39 years of age. Her primary issue was that she had not ovulated or had a period on her own since her 20s. After almost a year of weekly acupuncture treatments, she came in one day to announce her positive pregnancy test.

> We were both in shock because her period had never resumed. Rather, she spontaneously ovulated and got pregnant immediately. Debbie came back for help to have her second child because she didn't have a normal menstrual cycle when breastfeeding stopped. Again, she got pregnant after a few months of treatment without a period.

Acupuncture for POI

Used for thousands of years in China, acupuncture is an ancient option that is backed by modern science.

A pilot study of 31 women with POI followed their results in response to three months of acupuncture treatment given three times per week. The results showed increased estrogen and decreased luteinizing hormone, the hormone that tells the ovaries to release a mature egg (changes in the right direction!). About 20% of the women resumed having periods.[8]

While not a miracle cure for everyone, acupuncture may be a very effective treatment for some women with POI with no negative side effects.

Make sure you are getting enough melatonin

Animal studies show that treatment with melatonin reduces oxidative stress in the follicles and changes the cell signaling. This allows the follicles to mature.[9]

Reducing blue light exposure at night by turning off your electronic devices increases melatonin levels. If that's not a realistic expectation, wearing blue-blocking glasses will help. One study showed participants who wore them for two weeks at night increased melatonin production by more than 50%.[10]

Melatonin supplements are also readily available over the counter.

<u>5 Steps You Can Take Today to Treat POI:</u>

o   Workout: *Try a moderate weight lifting workout at the gym. If you aren't a gym member, body weight exercises, such as pushups and squats are easy (and free!) to do at home.*

o   Schedule some lab tests: *The only way to know how well your thyroid is functioning is to get it tested, so call your doctor to schedule an appointment or order your own lab work online.*

o   Avoid smokers: *Make an effort to remove yourself from situations where people will be smoking around you. This may mean taking a walk during lunch instead of hanging out with coworkers who are smoking.*

o   Eat a healthy diet that includes plenty of folate: *Fix a salad for dinner tonight that includes organic dark leafy green veggies topped with grilled steak.*

o   Stimulate melatonin production: *Turn off your electronic devices and turn down the overhead lights for a couple of hours before bed. Reading a book using a table lamp or relaxing in a bathtub surrounded by candles is a great way to wind down before bed while increasing melatonin naturally.*

CHAPTER 4

Enhancing Your Egg Quality

When seeking help from a fertility specialist, many women are told that they have "old eggs" or "poor egg quality." This may bring to mind an image of shriveled up beans rolling around in your ovaries. But that is not the case.

As you age, your cells are more likely to become damaged. This is true for egg cells as well as all your other cells, like skin and hair. However, measures can be taken to protect your cells. You use sunscreen to prevent damage to your skin cells from UV rays. Similarly, your egg cells can be safeguarded from harm with simple lifestyle changes.

Some of this damage can occur when the DNA replicates as the egg cell matures and gets ready for ovulation. This results in abnormal chromosomes in an egg, preventing fertilization. Abnormal chromosomes are the root cause of problems with getting pregnant for *many* women as they age.

What exactly does "egg quality" mean?

Every woman, no matter their age, has a percentage of abnormal egg cells, but that percentage increases considerably after age 35.

When fertility doctors and researchers talk about "poor egg quality," they are usually referring to the chromosomal abnormalities in older egg cells.

How do I know my egg quality?

Currently, no test can measure egg quality directly. This isn't something that you can quantify as with ovarian reserve or hormone levels.

Instead, age is the best predictor of problems with egg quality. That is why it is even more important as you age to do everything you can to prevent poor egg quality.

Chromosomes duplicate and divide to form the egg cell before ovulation

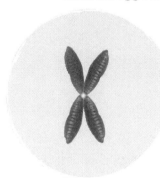 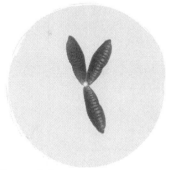

Normal chromosome   Abnormal chromosomes cause poor
                           egg quality and decreased fertility.

Doctors have a tendency to hyperfocus on chromosomal damage as it relates to egg quality. However, taking a more holistic view, you can enhance the overall health of the egg cell.

When we talk about improving egg quality:

- Some solutions will **improve the odds of having an egg with normal DNA.**

- Some solutions will also **enhance the health and quality of the egg cell.**

> ### Mary's Story
>
> At 43 years, Mary came to me to prepare for her third IVF cycle after two failed attempts. She wanted to do everything she could to improve her chances since it would be her last IVF due to finances.
>
> Based on her disappointing response to her previous IVF cycles, I encouraged her to wait until she had done some preparation.
>
> Although impatient to start her cycle because she felt she didn't have time to wait at 42 years of age, she heeded my advice and implemented my recommendations for six months.
>
> The results of her third (and final) cycle of IVF, as compared to her first two improved significantly with more eggs retrieved, higher fertilization rate, and enough frozen embryos for multiple transfers.
>
> In fact, she was able to get pregnant with not just one baby but another one two years later with an embryo from that same cycle.

How long does it take to improve egg quality?

Egg quality cannot be fixed after you ovulate. Instead, you need to prevent the DNA damage.

This isn't a quick fix but rather a way to improve the follicle cells before they develop into the final egg cell for ovulation.

The window for improving egg quality is two to four months before ovulation. This is the time when the follicle cells are developing, and the cell is getting ready to divide to form the egg cell that will end up being ovulated.

At birth, your body initially had millions of egg cells, but most of them will not develop into egg cells for ovulation.

The cell that goes on to become the ovulated one needs to be optimized, so it can be the very best, healthiest cell possible.

Egg Cell Development Timeline

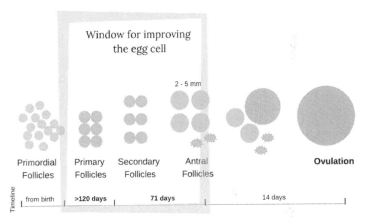

It is important to do everything you can to stack the odds towards a better quality egg and improving your chances of conceiving.

Start now, but expect the results a few months down the road.

How can I improve my egg quality naturally?

Research shows the actions you can take to help improve egg quality are all things that enhance overall health. These include:

- **Lengthening your telomeres**. These caps at the end of your DNA protect the delicate strands from damage. Lengthening your telomeres can slow down the aging process at the DNA level.

- **Adding the right antioxidants.** Reducing oxidative stress in the follicles can help to prevent DNA damage to the egg.

- **Getting rid of toxicants that cause damage**. The toxicants that you are exposed to on a daily basis, such as BPA, parabens, and phthalates, all have been shown to impact fertility. To maximize your chances to conceive, limit your exposure to these chemicals.[1]

- **Improving your mitochondrial function**. Mitochondria are the powerhouse of your cells including your egg cells. They make the ATP that the egg cell uses for energy.

- **Focusing on sleep and melatonin production**. Sleep and melatonin are also critical to healthy egg cells. Melatonin acts as an antioxidant in the egg, preventing damage to the cell from harmful molecules. A healthy sleep schedule can help with maintaining your overall health and the health of your developing egg cells.[2]

To maximize the improvement in egg quality, *all* of the above are important.

If you take a multifactorial approach rather than a singular one, you will get better results. For example, adding a supplement and ignoring the other strategies will limit your improvement.

THE TAKEAWAY MESSAGE IS:
GET HEALTHY TO GET PREGNANT.

These next sections and chapters explore the science of why egg quality matters and then outline the lifestyle changes that will make the most impact.

Telomeres and egg quality

Your cells are dividing all the time, replicating their DNA and creating new cells as the old ones wear out.

Think about your skin cells. You lose dead skin every day, and new skin cells take their place.

When your body creates new cells, the DNA inside the nucleus is copied. All 46 of your chromosomes get duplicated so that your new cell has the same genes as the parent cell.

At the end of each chromosome is a telomere, which acts as a cap, kind of like the end of a shoelace. The telomere keeps the end of the chromosome safe from replication errors. It also keeps the chromosomes from accidentally sticking together.

The cells in your body can replicate many times before the telomeres at the end get too short. Once the cells have reached that limit, though, they end up going through senescence or cell death.

Oxidative stress in the cells can also shorten the telomeres. Oxidative stress results from having too much free radicals causing damage to the cells. Excessive free radicals can come from your environment including fried foods, alcohol, tobacco smoke, pesticides, air pollutants, and X-Rays.

Your egg cells haven't been undergoing a bunch of cell division before ovulation. The eggs start out as primordial follicles that haven't been replicating. While they only go through a couple of cell divisions, the replication must be perfect for a quality egg.

Thus, oxidative stress in the follicles can result in abnormal chromosome division. Egg quality decreases, and infertility increases.

What causes shorter telomeres?

Studies show that increased reactive oxygen species (ROS) in the cell cause oxidative damage. This is the main cause of telomere shortening in the egg cells. Various environmental stresses lead to excessive production of ROS causing progressive oxidative damage.[3]

How do short telomeres affect fertility?

Shortened telomeres could be at the heart of infertility as you age. In fact, some researchers think this is the main cause of infertility in aging. Chromosomal abnormalities and poor egg quality are a direct result of short telomeres.[4]

Your genes also play a role in how long your telomeres are. Some people carry genetic variants that are associated with shorter telomeres. Others have variants that cause longer telomeres.

Research directly links shorter telomeres to chromosomal errors. Mothers with shorter telomeres are more likely to have errors in the processes by which the chromosomes replicate and divide. This leads to a higher rate of Down syndrome in egg cells with shorter telomeres.[5]

Lifestyle choices can shorten your telomeres

Here are some studies on how lifestyle choices affect telomere length:

- A study of Indian women undergoing ART found that tobacco use may shorten telomeres.[6] Other studies confirm this result. Exposure to cigarette smoke shortens telomeres.[7]

- A sedentary lifestyle may cause shorter telomeres. In fact, women who were sedentary had shorter telomeres equal to 4.4 years of aging.[8]

- Not sleeping enough or having poor quality sleep may shorten telomeres.[9]

- Staying up too late is also associated with shorter telomere length.[10]

- Drinking sugar-sweetened beverages, such as soda, may cause shorter telomere length.[11]

- A lack of fiber in the diet connects to shorter telomere length.[12]

- The ratio of omega-6 to omega-3 fats in the diet is important to telomere length. A higher omega-6 to omega-3 may shorten telomere length.[13]

Dana's Story

Dana was a daily smoker for the past 10 of her 38 years. Although she knew she needed to stop before getting pregnant, she had difficulty quitting because her husband and social circle all smoked. The effects of smoking were evident on her prematurely lined face and deep crow's feet.

After trying to conceive naturally without success for two years, she sought medical help. Her fertility doctors recommended IVF due to diminished ovarian reserve. In preparation, she sought my guidance.

Given her long history, I recommended she delay her IVF for at least six months to give her body time to recover from the effects of smoking. Over the course of the next few months, she gradually reduced her daily cigarette consumption to complete abstinence.

Her IVF was a success – a testament to her dedication to living a cleaner and healthier lifestyle.

What can I do to lengthen my telomeres?

Your body produces an enzyme called telomerase that can add to the end of telomeres and lengthen them.

Telomerase is naturally active in stem cells and some immune cells. So what can you do to increase telomerase?

Supplemental melatonin increases telomerase in an animal study. The study showed that melatonin increased telomere length and the number of viable egg cells.[14] One more reason to focus on sleep! Blocking blue light at night from TV, cell phones, and laptops can increase melatonin.

Astragalus, a traditional Chinese medicine herb, may help lengthen telomeres. Several clinical trials show astragalus components can lengthen telomeres by activating telomerase. Besides lengthening telomeres, it is also anti-inflammatory.[15]

5 natural ways to lengthen your telomeres to improve egg quality and reduce DNA damage:

o *Eliminate sugar sweetened beverages. Swap out your daily soda for an herbal tea.*

o *Get active. You don't have to go out and jog five miles every day. Moderate activity is enough to lengthen telomeres.*

o *Increase your intake of omega-3 fats by eating mercury-safe fish. Decrease your consumption of omega-6 fats by cutting out fried foods.*

o *Make sure you are getting enough fiber in your diet. Replace refined carbohydrates (bread, pasta, and packaged foods) with whole foods instead.*

o *Sleep well. Go to bed at a reasonable hour and focus on getting quality sleep.*

Antioxidants for preventing DNA damage and improving egg quality

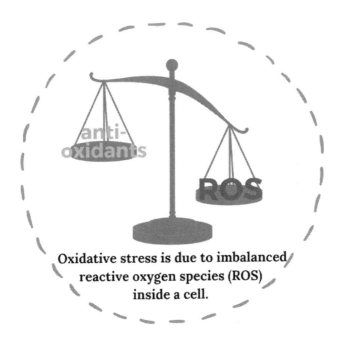

Oxidative stress is due to imbalanced reactive oxygen species (ROS) inside a cell.

One way that egg quality declines as we age is through an excess amount of oxidative stress.

You've probably heard that antioxidants are good for you. Vitamin C from fruits and vegetables or vitamin E from nuts usually come to mind when you think of antioxidants from foods.

But do antioxidants really work to improve egg quality? Some studies show that they do work, and other studies show that taking a handful of antioxidant supplements is ineffective.

Let's dig into the science and figure out what is going on in the ovaries and which antioxidants may work to boost fertility.

Oxidative stress in the ovaries

Oxidative stress occurs when the cells have too many oxidants (or reactive oxygen species) and not enough antioxidants. This can lead to damage within the cell and can be a cause of decreased egg quality.[16]

The reactive oxygen species (ROS) within a cell have positive effects but only if the ROS is balanced with the body's natural antioxidant system.

What causes oxidative stress?

We are all exposed to a fairly high burden of environmental toxicants each day through breathing in air pollutants, putting parabens (chemical preservatives widely used in cosmetic products) on our skin, consuming foods sprayed with pesticides, and more. This environmental exposure combines with a natural decrease in antioxidants as we age to increase oxidative stress in our cells, including our egg cells.

Another cause of increased oxidative stress is insulin resistance. Studies show that insulin resistance, or higher fasting blood glucose levels, increase oxidative stress and cause mitochondrial dysfunction in the egg cells.[17] This may be why pregnancy rates are lower in women with pre-diabetes and diabetes.[18]

> ### Belinda's Story
>
> At 40 years, Belinda was overweight, bordering on obese. Her blood glucose and hemoglobin A1c levels were at pre-diabetic levels. Almost daily, she had fast food with her coworkers for lunch. Dinner time was usually take out in front of the TV. She felt she was too busy to cook meals. I told her that she needed to choose her priority – baby or fast food.
>
> She chose baby.

Although initially with difficulty, she consistently implemented my recommendations. Over the course of our two years together, she was rewarded with a gradual weight loss that was sustainable. At 42 years, she finally conceived a healthy baby.

How does oxidative stress decrease egg quality?

A recent study determined that lower oxidative stress within the fluid of the follicles directly related to better outcomes in women undergoing IVF. This is an important study because it showed exactly how oxidative stress decreases fertility.[19]

You may be thinking—just give me a bunch of antioxidant pills. Let's get rid of oxidative stress in the ovaries. Well, it may not work quite that simply.

How do antioxidants from foods work?

The polyphenols in fruits, vegetables, wine, and tea are often called antioxidants, but that is an oversimplification. In reality, many of the natural polyphenols from foods act as pro-oxidants in the body. They cause your body to stimulate its built-in antioxidant system.

What are these antioxidants that your body produces? Glutathione is an important one for quenching the overabundance of oxidative stress in the cell. Superoxide dismutase, or SOD, and catalase are two more antioxidants that your body makes. All of these are important in preventing oxidative stress within the egg cells.[20]

The goal then is to boost the body's natural production of antioxidants. Among these, boosting glutathione may have the biggest impact.

Can glutathione increase fertility?

Studies of couples undergoing IVF show that higher glutathione levels are linked to a greater chance of conceiving.[21] Additionally, animal studies show that adding glutathione improves egg cells that have been damaged due to oxidative stress.[22]

Glutathione is made in the body using the amino acids glutamate, cysteine, and glycine. Meats, bone broth, and vegetables are good sources of these amino acids.

The supplement N-acetyl cysteine (NAC) is a good source of cysteine if you aren't getting enough from your diet. NAC supplements have been shown to boost the body's production of glutathione.[23]

You can also supplement with glutathione directly.

A word of caution...

While you want to boost your antioxidant status enough to bring oxidative stress into balance, you don't want to go overboard and decrease ROS too much.

ROS is necessary as a signaling molecule in cells and is important for conception in the right amount. Huge amounts of antioxidants (way more than you could get from foods or standard supplements) have been shown in rat studies to decrease fertility.[24]

Boosting Nrf2 for fertility

At the heart of the body's antioxidant defense system lies the Nrf2 pathway. Nuclear factor erythroid 2-related factor 2, or Nrf2, is your body's master regulator of antioxidant defense.

Nrf2 controls the production of over 200 proteins that protect your cells from oxidative stress.

How does this work? Too much ROS in the cell prompts Nrf2 to move into the cell nucleus. There, it activates the production of your body's antioxidant enzymes.

Too little Nrf2 activity causes an imbalance in the cell, leading to oxidative stress. Studies show that low Nrf2 can cause chronic diseases, such as type 2 diabetes and heart disease.[25]

What is oxidative stress?

An imbalance between pro-oxidants (ROS) and antioxidants in the cell leads to oxidative stress. This happens when ROS production is greater than the antioxidant system can handle.

What exactly is ROS? It is a general term for reactive molecules, such as hydrogen peroxide and superoxide.

Your mitochondria naturally produce ROS as a byproduct of energy production. Your cells can also produce ROS when breaking down toxins. Thus, too many toxins can lead to oxidative stress in the cells.

ROS in the right amounts, though, can act as a signaling molecule in the cell. The goal is to keep it in balance rather than to eliminate it completely.

Too much can cause damage, but some ROS is necessary.

How does Nrf2 affect fertility?

As the follicle cell develops into the egg cell ready for ovulation, ROS plays an important role. While too much ROS damages the egg cell, there are periods during egg cell development when ROS acts as a signaling molecule.

Oxidative stress is tightly regulated in the ovaries. As the follicle cell develops into the mature egg cell, a lot of energy is needed from the mitochondria. In turn, this produces a high level of ROS. The ROS then causes activation of the body's antioxidant system through the Nrf2 pathway.[26]

Studies show that too much oxidative stress plays a role in infertility in women and men. Our modern world is full of stress and environmental toxin exposure. Thus, the balance is almost always tipped towards too much ROS instead of too much on the antioxidant side.[27]

The key is to activate the Nrf2 signaling pathway so that your body naturally balances out the excess oxidative stress.

What happens without enough Nrf2? Animal studies show that stopping the Nrf2 signal will stop the development of an egg cell prior to ovulation. We definitely don't want that![28]

Other studies show that activating the Nrf2 pathway delays age-associated fertility problems.[29]

A number of other studies show the importance of balancing oxidative stress and activating the Nrf2 pathway. This is true for the development of the egg cell and for the growing baby.[30]

How can I increase Nrf2?

There are several ways to safely raise Nrf2 when trying to conceive.

First, regular exercise increases ROS, which then enhances Nrf2 production. The key here is regular exercise.

A sudden spurt of hard exercise will boost Nrf2 in response to the ROS produced in the mitochondria. But you don't just want a short increase in Nrf2 in the muscles. Instead, moderate exercise that is done regularly stimulates Nrf2 throughout the body in anticipation of more exercise tomorrow.[31]

Next, there are natural plant polyphenols that can raise Nrf2.

Curcumin, which is found in the spice turmeric, increases the Nrf2 signal and decreases oxidative stress in the egg cell.[32] You can take curcumin as a supplement (best absorbed with piperine included), or you can liberally use turmeric in your cooking.

Citrus fruits contain naringenin, which has also been shown to raise Nrf2 levels. An animal study showed that raising Nrf2 levels has therapeutic potential to treat endometriosis.[33]

Broccoli is a rich source of sulforaphane, which is a potent activator of Nrf2.[34] Broccoli sprouts have the highest amounts of sulforaphane and are great to use in a smoothie or to take as a supplement.

A diet rich in olive oil increases Nrf2. The polyphenols in olive oil decrease oxidative stress in the cells.[35]

3 Steps you can take today to boost Nrf2 for antioxidant defense:

- o *Making time to exercise regularly is important for fertility in many ways. Get into a routine of getting moderate exercise every day. This can be as simple as changing where you park so that you get in a 15-minute brisk walk to and from work. Or you could get some weights and resistance bands to use for a half hour each evening while watching Netflix.*

- o *If your diet isn't abundant in polyphenol-rich foods, you may want to consider supplementing. Try adding curcumin, sulforaphane, or naringenin. While you don't want to go overboard with high doses of antioxidant supplements, most people will benefit from adding antioxidants.*

- o *Even if you choose to supplement, adding foods, such as broccoli and olive oil, are easy ways to boost your Nrf2 and balance your diet. Focus on getting fresh vegetables in your diet each day, and choose organic whenever possible.*

CHAPTER 5

Getting Rid of the Toxicants that Decrease the Quality of Your Eggs

Our modern world is filled with conveniences to make our lives easier. Plastic containers to store our food, pans coated with Teflon for easy cleaning, and pesticides to keep our homes free of critters.

But these conveniences may come at a price to your fertility.

Research on common toxicants shows a clear association with your ability to get pregnant.

A quick note on terminology . . . Technically, a toxin is a natural product, such as a poison from a plant or bacteria. A toxicant is a synthetic or man-made substance that is toxic.

Endocrine disrupting chemicals, such as BPA and phthalates, are everywhere.

We are all exposed each day to an array of endocrine-disrupting chemicals that abound in our modern environment.

Connie's Story

Trying to maintain her composure, Connie shared with me her seven-year struggle to get pregnant. At 44 years old, she didn't know what else to do.

Using donor eggs was out of the question because of the high cost. She had already done three IVF cycles with no success.

Her days were consumed with the desire to have a baby but tinged with the fear that it was too late. She spent a lot of time on the internet reading blogs on how to improve fertility and joining forums to see what other women were doing. Trying to figure a solution resulted in sleepless nights. She was exhausted, worried, and frustrated.

My first recommendation to her was to stop researching on the internet. As long as she was working with me, I would be her primary resource for fertility, guiding her through the next steps.

Placing the responsibility of improving her fertility on me, she slept better and was less anxious throughout the day. With more energy, she started to exercise several times a week consistently. She replaced many of her personal care and cleaning products with less toxic alternatives. She paid a lot of attention to being as healthy as she could be, physically and emotionally.

After more than a year of diligent attention to her well-being, she finally had a healthy baby.

What is an endocrine disruptor?

The endocrine system consists of glands that secrete the hormones which control growth, reproduction, mood, and metabolism. This includes your ovaries, thyroid, adrenals, and the hormones that affect reproduction.

An endocrine disruptor is a substance that you take into your body which binds to one of your body's hormone receptors and modifies the way your natural hormones work.

Almost everyone is exposed to endocrine disruptors on a daily basis. Examples include BPA, phthalates, dioxins, and genistein. All of these can alter your reproductive hormones, decreasing your ability to get pregnant.

Fertility doctors and researchers define poor egg quality in terms of having DNA abnormalities, such as too many or too few chromosomes. This causes a decrease in fertility due to the eggs not being able to be fertilized.

Toxicants that are endocrine disruptors can increase the risk of infertility in several ways, including altering reproductive hormone levels and causing harm to the egg.

A recent review of endocrine disruptors sums up the issue:[1]

- *Endocrine disruptors affect the ovaries, causing decreased antral follicle count and premature ovarian insufficiency.*

- *BPA exposure has been specifically linked in multiple studies to egg quality, and phthalates are linked with hormonal changes.*

Let's get down and dirty with the science and then discuss steps you can take today to solve these problems.

Bisphenols (BPA and BPS) decrease fertility

BPA (bisphenol-A) was first manufactured in the 1930s. Since then, it has become a common part of our daily lives. BPA is a plasticizer that is found in many common products, including plastic kitchen containers, canned foods, thermal printed receipts, canned beverages, and toys.

In 2008, several studies came out that made headlines about the concerns with BPA, especially in children's products. Many states passed laws banning BPA in teething rings and baby. In response, manufacturers started producing BPA-Free plastics due to consumer demands.

BPS (bisphenol-S) is an alternative used to replace BPA. But this isn't necessarily a better solution.

Studies on the bisphenols, including BPS, that have been produced to replace BPA show that they also have negative effects on reproductive hormones.[2] In fact, one study that examined multiple different kinds of commonly used household plastics found that most of the plastics leached endocrine disruptors, even the ones marketed as BPA Free.[3]

Animal studies show that bisphenols from plastics cause various reproductive problems, including premature ovarian insufficiency.[4]

One study concluded that lifelong exposure to low levels of BPA "reduces fertility with age." The fact that this study used low levels of BPA is important. These are the levels that we are exposed to every day.[5]

Another animal study found that increasing levels of BPA directly reduced the number of offspring. One way that it reduced fertility was through impairing the implantation of the embryo in the uterus.

Mice chewing on plastic in cages that contained BPA prompted another study. It was noted that the mice had fewer normal egg cells when they had consumed BPA. The researchers then gave a group of mice low levels of BPA to measure and check the results. These mice also had decreased egg quality due to changes in the chromosomes of the eggs.[6]

To put it simply, animal studies clearly show that BPA decreases egg quality by inducing chromosomal changes.

Human studies on BPA show a variety of different results. Epidemiological studies use large population groups to see if there is an effect from a toxicant. These studies are often difficult when it comes to things that everyone in the population is exposed to. Some epidemiological studies find that BPA may have no impact on overall fertility rates, but a meta-analysis that looked at several studies concludes that "BPA is an ovarian, uterine, and prostate toxicant at a level below . . . the proposed safe level."[7]

Let me say that again:

BPA is a toxicant that is affecting the ovaries at levels we are exposed to every day.

Specific research studies on women with infertility also point to an impact from BPA.

- A study on women undergoing IVF found that as BPA levels increased, the number of good eggs available for retrieval decreased.[8]

- An overview of research on infertility due to endocrine-disrupting chemicals states that BPA binds to the estrogen receptors and decreases the production of reproductive hormones.[9]

Practical ways to decrease your BPA and BPS levels

Plastics are everywhere, and they make life easier but some simple steps will help you drastically reduce the amount of BPA you are exposed to each day. Let's take a look at where the BPA is coming from and how your body detoxifies it.

How quickly can your body get rid of BPA?

It is important to know how long it will take to get the BPA out of your system. BPA is metabolized by the body fairly quickly. In adults it usually takes 3 to 24 hours to break down and eliminate BPA. It does accumulate in adipose (fat) tissue, so sudden weight loss may release more BPA into your body.

Taking steps today to decrease BPA exposure could have an immediate effect on your reproductive hormones and fertility.

Can anything help to reduce the effects of BPA?

Melatonin, which your body produces in great quantities when it is dark outside, has been shown in animal studies to specifically reverse the effects of BPA on oocytes.[10]

This is a huge reason to prioritize your evening routine and your sleep! Light in the blue wavelengths at night, such as from TVs, cell phones, and computers, reduce the amount of melatonin that your body produces. Blocking out that blue light, either by wearing blue light-blocking glasses or by turning off electronics and bright overhead lights, will allow your melatonin levels to naturally rise at the right time. Additionally, you may want to consider a low-dose, time-release melatonin supplement if you have poor quality sleep.

Where is all this BPA (and BPS) coming from?

Canned foods and condiments are a big source of BPA in people's diets. A study of food in the United States found that 75% of the 267 food items sampled contained BPA or a similar bisphenol. The highest amounts were found in foods that were packaged in cans and condiments since the linings of the cans often contain BPA. Lowest amounts of BPA were found in fruits, which are usually unpackaged.[11]

Another study found BPA in 73% of canned products. But only 7% of non-canned foods had BPA in them.[12] Stick with fresh and frozen vegetables!

Both BPA and BPS can leach from plastic water bottles or coffee cups, especially if they get hot or contain hot drinks. Reusable plastic water bottles that aren't marked as BPA and BPS free usually contain one of the bisphenols. Aluminum drinking bottles that are lined with epoxy resin may also contain BPA in the lining. Look for glass water bottles or aluminum bottles without a lining.

Fast food items often contain more BPA than items that you cook at home. The paper or cardboard food wrappers often contain BPA in their coating. In general, people who often eat

45

out or order take-out have higher BPA levels than those who cook at home.[13]

5 action steps you can take today to reduce your BPA levels:

o *Reduce or completely eliminate canned foods. Switch to fresh or frozen fruits and vegetables.*

o *Switch from plastic water bottles to glass or stainless steel bottles.*

o *Cook at home more often. Plan ahead and have some simple meal options, such as vegetables and meat to put on the grill.*

o *Get 8 to 9 hours of quality sleep and let your melatonin levels rise naturally at night. Blocking out the blue light from electronics and bright overhead lights at night will increase your melatonin levels, protecting your eggs from BPA.*

o *Stop storing and microwaving your leftovers in plastic, including Styrofoam and lined cardboard boxes. It is time to start collecting glass containers of various sizes to store your hot food.*

Phthalates: plastics, make up, fragrances, and nail polish

Joy's Story

For as long as she could remember, Joy had experienced inexplicable fatigue. At 22 years old, she was diagnosed with chronic fatigue syndrome. She had difficulty keeping jobs because she had called in sick so often. Since being married, she was fortunate that she could stay at home to take care of her health. She also complained of brain fog and poor memory.

After hearing her symptoms, I advised her to discard all personal care and household products that weren't essential and choose natural, chemical free options.

Immediately, she started feeling more energy and was clear headed. She had never used birth control during her five years of marriage. Within six months of working with me, she was pregnant.

Phthalates are a class of chemicals commonly found in and around us daily. They are used as plasticizers and found in some plastics. Phthalates are often used in artificial fragrances, such as in air fresheners or laundry products. They add to the flexibility and durability in nail polish. For many women, much of their daily exposure comes from the phthalates added to cosmetics and personal care products.

We are exposed to phthalates through ingesting them, absorbing them, and inhaling them. Our body then breaks them down, or metabolizes, and excretes the phthalates through urine or stool.

Almost every adult in the U.S. and most of the developed world has metabolites of phthalates in their urine or blood every day. It is truly ubiquitous in our modern world.

But are phthalates really a problem? Research clearly shows that phthalates act as an endocrine disruptor to harm fertility and the quality of your eggs.

Studies show that higher phthalate exposure decreases fertility:

- A study of 187 women undergoing IVF in the U.S. found that higher concentrations of phthalate metabolites in their urine corresponded to a lower number of oocytes (egg cells) retrieved and decreased oocyte maturity. Both of these factors decrease the chance that IVF will work.[14]

- A review of studies on how phthalates affect fertility in IVF clearly showed that higher phthalate levels (metabolites in urine) correlated to decreased number of quality eggs and fewer total and fertilized eggs.[15]

- Phthalates have been shown to impact progesterone and estradiol levels, key reproductive hormones when trying to conceive.[16]

- Animal studies clearly show how phthalate exposure affects antral follicle count, decreasing the number of pregnancies.[17]

- Six hundred women undergoing IVF and their male partners found that higher levels of phthalates per couple caused a significant decrease in pregnancy outcomes. This study is a good reminder that phthalate exposure also impacts male fertility.[18]

- Higher exposure to phthalates is also linked to a 60% increase in miscarriage risk.[19]

How are you exposed to phthalates on a daily basis?

Phthalate exposure can come by eating foods that contain phthalate residue, inhaling phthalate particles, or absorption through skin exposure.

Cosmetics, lotions, hair care products, nail polish, shampoo, and fragrances all can contain phthalates. One study found that most of these products contain some kind of phthalate, including products marketed for baby care.[20]

Reading the labels is important, but confusing. There are many types of phthalates in personal care products. Take the time to read the labels on products you use regularly. Look for terms such as dibutyl phthalate, butyl benzyl phthalate, DEP, DBP, DEHP, and fragrance.

Vinyl shower curtains and other vinyl products can also give off phthalates, which you can breathe in during a hot shower. Consider switching to a fabric shower curtain.

Similar to BPA, household dust often contains phthalates. This is one good reason to get out a damp rag and clean off the fan blades and baseboards regularly.

How can you decrease the harmful effects of phthalates?

While reducing exposure is very important, you will likely have some exposure to phthalates.

The good news is that some manufacturers are reducing their use of phthalates due to consumer concerns.

Getting enough folate may also help decrease the negative effects of phthalates.

A study of pregnant women examined their phthalate metabolite levels during their first trimester. This was compared with the time it took them to get pregnant. Higher phthalate and BPA levels corresponded with longer time to conception, but supplementing with folate eliminated this increase. Folate is important for many reasons when trying to conceive a healthy baby, and its role in counteracting the effects of phthalates is another one.[21]

5 action steps you can take today to reduce phthalate exposure:

o Check your laundry detergent, fabric softener, and dryer sheets. These often contain artificial fragrances that increase your phthalate exposure. Switch to a natural laundry option that is labeled "free and clear" or contains essential oils for fragrance.

o Add more folate to your diet. Grass-fed beef liver is a great source of folate and other essential vitamins. A 100g serving of liver packs a whopping 212 mcg of folate. Not a liver fan? Eat more dark, leafy green vegetables. Take a methylfolate supplement to ensure adequate levels—800 mcg a day is recommended.

- o Go through your cosmetics, hair care products, and lotions. Read the ingredients to see if they contain phthalates. Find replacements for the items that contain ingredients that are likely to be impacting your fertility.

- o Get rid of the artificial air fresheners around your house and workspace.

- o Break out the dust rag and clean up any household dust that may contain phthalates and BPA.

Parabens in your personal care products

Parabens, prevalent in personal care products, are another source of endocrine-disrupting chemicals. They are used in many products as an antimicrobial agent to prevent mold or bacteria build up.

Parabens are found in products such as:

- Toothpaste

- Deodorant

- Shampoo

- Conditioner

- Lotion

- Sunscreen

- Cosmetics

- Foods

If the ingredients label contains the words methylparaben, ethylparaben, propylparaben, butylparaben, or isobutylparaben, then the product contains parabens.

In 2014, the European Union banned five types of parabens for use in cosmetics.

At this time, the U.S. and Canada have no restrictions on parabens in personal care products.

Do parabens decrease fertility?

One study reports that couples who have higher amounts of paraben metabolites in their body had a decreased fertility rate—by 34%. This is a measurable impact on fertility that can't be ignored.[22]

Another study looked at the impact of parabens on ovarian reserve. The study showed that women with higher propylparaben concentrations trended towards lower antral follicle counts (lower ovarian reserve).[23]

The good news here is that parabens are eliminated from the body fairly quickly. So, stopping your exposure to parabens will allow them to leave your body within a few days.

> ### 2 action steps you can take today to reduce paraben exposure:
>
> o   Check labels on your personal care products, especially lotions, cosmetics, and sunscreens. Swap out the ones that contain parabens for more natural options. This is a great time to clean out and eliminate all of the personal care products you no longer need. In addition, consider minimizing the number of products you use on your skin and hair.
>
> o   Consider switching to a natural deodorant. Not only will you avoid the parabens, but many deodorants also contain phthalates as part of the fragrance.

CHAPTER 6

Improving Mitochondrial Function in Your Eggs

Mitochondria are known as the *powerhouses* of cells. They convert the food that you eat into the energy that your body uses. They're the *engine* of your eggs.

Most cells in your body have hundreds of mitochondria in them. As your egg cells mature, going from a microscopic primordial follicle cell to a visible egg cell, mitochondria multiply exponentially to 100,000–500,000 or more in fully mature eggs. There are more mitochondria in one egg cell than in any other cell in the body!

The reason for this staggering increase is because the egg is actively preparing itself for the increased energy demands of successful fertilization and eventual embryo development.

Unfortunately, as you age, the number and efficiency of mitochondria decline. This happens to both women and men in all cells, not just the eggs. This decrease is a result of aging, so it's not unique to your situation.

When it comes to reproduction, though, men don't need to worry as much about mitochondria in the sperm cells. While the egg cell is working hard to create up to a half a million mitochondria, the sperm cell only has a couple of hundred. Once fertilization occurs, the fertilized egg actually destroys the mitochondria from the sperm. Only mom's mitochondria survive and are inherited by the baby.

Before ovulation, the egg cell is attached to the wall of the ovary. If it is fertilized and becomes an embryo, it reconnects to your body after implantation.

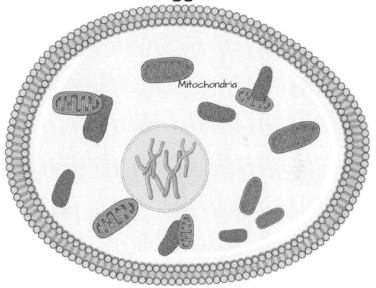

Mitochondria produce the energy that the egg cell needs.

Mitochondria

An egg cell can have up to 500,000 mitochondria in it!

This means that during the window between ovulation and implantation (up to 7 days), the embryo is free floating. It is dependent on energy produced by the existing mitochondria in the egg at the moment of ovulation. More mitochondria are made only after the fertilized embryo implants into the uterus.

Studies show that one of the disadvantages of older eggs is that they tend to be a little smaller and have fewer mitochondria than eggs from younger women. The shape and function of some of the mitochondria in older eggs has also been shown to be dysfunctional. This causes a decrease in the energy produced by the mitochondria.

The older egg might have just enough mitochondria and, therefore, energy to allow for fertilization and the initial stages of embryonic development. However, if there isn't a surplus of mitochondria, the embryo will run out of "juice" and have problems with development before implantation can be achieved.

To increase the egg quality so that fertilization and implantation of a healthy embryo can occur, you need to increase the number and improve the efficiency of the mitochondria. In fact, research shows that adding more mitochondria to the egg cell improves IVF outcomes.[1]

To have healthy mitochondria, your cells need all the building blocks for producing adenosine triphosphate (ATP), the molecule which provides energy for all of the cells' processes. This includes plenty of vitamins, such as riboflavin (B2) and niacin (B3). Your mitochondria also need minerals and nutrients, such as magnesium, iron, manganese, and CoQ10.

Studies in animals show that a low protein diet specifically causes damage to the mitochondria in the egg cell.[2] Getting plenty of protein from a variety of sources is important in the weeks leading up to conception.

Mitochondrial function decreases with age due in part to oxidative stress. All the things discussed in the previous chapter on egg quality apply here. Healthy mitochondria are part of a healthy egg, and inherent in this is a balance of oxidative stress.[3] Getting plenty of antioxidant rich foods in your diet is important.

Insulin resistance is a specific cause of oxidative stress in the egg cells. Insulin resistance occurs when your body stops responding to the hormone insulin it produces and no longer uses glucose efficiently. Risk factors for developing insulin resistance include being overweight, a sedentary lifestyle, smoking, and poor sleeping habits.

Studies in animals show that insulin resistance impacts the mitochondrial function of the egg cell through increasing oxidative stress. Your preconception diet is important not only for the nutrients it provides but also for stabilizing your insulin levels. This is one more reason to reduce sugar and processed carbohydrates to keep the mitochondria in the egg cell healthy!

Research-backed ways to improve mitochondrial function

Here are some research-backed actions you can take today to improve your mitochondrial function and your egg quality.

Avoid taking medications that damage your mitochondria. Acetaminophen, NSAIDs, some antibiotics, illegal drugs, statins, and L-Dopa have all been shown to damage mitochondrial function. Of course, talk to your doctor about any prescribed medications before you stop them. If you are taking NSAIDs or acetaminophen daily for inflammation, this is the time to figure out the root cause of the inflammation and do whatever you can to reduce your daily intake of anti-inflammatories.

Giving your mitochondria the fuel that they need is vitally important. Protein and folate are both essential for mitochondrial health in the developing egg cell. Omega-3 fatty acids, such as from fish oil, are also important for your mitochondria.

Building muscle mass increases ATP production in the mitochondria. Studies show the benefit of moderate, regular exercise for increasing mitochondrial function.[4]

CoQ10 is important for mitochondrial function in the egg cells. In animal studies, ensuring enough CoQ10 has been shown to reverse age-related mitochondrial decline in egg cells.[5]

If you aren't getting enough of the nutrients needed for mitochondrial function from your diet, quality supplements can fill in the gaps. Supplements that have been shown to improve mitochondrial function include CoQ10, NAC, and magnesium.[6]

5 Steps you can take today to boost mitochondrial function:

o Make sure you are getting enough CoQ10 in your diet. Foods rich in CoQ10 include organ meats, such as heart and liver, and meats, such as beef and pork. If you aren't getting enough CoQ10 in your diet, consider supplementing.

o Grab your headphones, put on a podcast or some music, and get outside for some exercise today. Moderate, regular exercise will help to increase mitochondrial function.

o Have fatty fish like wild salmon, herring, mackerel, or sardines several times a week. Fish are a great source of both protein and omega-3 fatty acids.

o Go through your medicine cabinet to see if any of the OTC medications you take regularly could be affecting your mitochondria.

o Cut back on sugar and processed carbohydrates to stabilize your insulin levels. Replace sodas and sugar-sweetened drinks with herbal teas and purified water.

CHAPTER 7

Sleep and Melatonin: A Key to Conception

Everyone knows that sleep is important for good health, and it is also very important when trying to conceive. Getting enough quality sleep is something that you need to prioritize at this time in your life.

Let's get into the details of why sleep is important and how it enhances your fertility odds.

The importance of sleep can be attributed, in part, to melatonin.

Melatonin levels rise at night while you sleep. It is often thought of as a *sleep hormone*, but melatonin actually does a lot in your body!

Melatonin acts in several specific ways to help the reproductive cycle.

In a nutshell, melatonin:

- Acts as an antioxidant within the egg cell, improving egg quality.

- Acts as a signaling molecule in the brain, controlling reproductive hormone rhythm.

- Acts within the uterus, protecting the embryo and facilitating implantation.

Ana's Story

A newlywed, Ana came to me stressed out and worried that it might be too late for her to get pregnant at 43. She worked 10-hour days and often went in on the weekends. Although she loved her job, she was on the verge of burnout with little time for herself, husband, friends, and family. She went to bed late and rose early because she worked so much.

My first suggestion was to decrease her work day to eight hours as quickly as possible. She had to understand that she has the rest of her life to work, but her fertile window period is now. As a people pleaser, it was difficult for her to set her boundaries because she felt guilty for not doing more.

Over the weeks as she reduced her hours and freed up more time, I encouraged her to create a regular sleep schedule. It was obvious she wasn't getting enough sleep because she always woke up tired. Once she got a steady eight to nine hours of sleep every day, she felt like a new woman. She was happy, excited, relaxed, and much more confident about her fertility journey.

Over the next few months, she continued to make small adjustments to her lifestyle. I told her that her goal was to create a lifestyle that she enjoys and is satisfied with, where life is unfolding easily and naturally with little effort. In doing so, she would get aligned with her desire to have a child, and her happy ending came.

Melatonin as an antioxidant

As discussed previously, egg quality is vitally important, especially as you age.

One main factor affecting your egg quality is the production of reactive oxygen species (ROS) within the egg, specifically within the mitochondria of the egg cell.

This buildup of ROS is called oxidative stress and is a natural byproduct of aging so it can't be avoided. However, significant increases in ROS are often due to environmental toxins, like poor quality food, harmful lifestyle choices, chronic stress—basically, living in a modern-day society.

Several antioxidants protect your cells from the effects of ROS. *One of the most important and potent antioxidants your body produces naturally is melatonin.*

Melatonin is found at higher levels within the ovaries and the egg follicle as compared to the rest of the body. Within the egg, it neutralizes the damage from excess ROS.

Melatonin is a unique hormone in that it can pass easily through the outer membrane of the mitochondria, the power plant of the cell.

In addition to acting directly as an antioxidant within the mitochondria, melatonin also stimulates the body to create other natural antioxidants, such as glutathione, catalase, and superoxide dismutase (SOD). These antioxidants work together to protect the cell's nuclear DNA from damage (so important for egg cells!) as well as protecting other parts of the cell.

Not only can melatonin protect eggs from oxidative stress, it may actually speed the growth and maturation of ovarian follicles, according to promising preliminary animal studies.[1]

Melatonin and ovulation

The reproductive hormone cycles are both intricate and simply amazing. Women everywhere understand the monthly cycling

59

of hormone levels involved in menstruation. Your reproductive hormones also have a daily rhythm, rising and falling in concert over the course of 24 hours.

Melatonin regulates gonadotropin-releasing hormone (GnRH), one of the key players in your reproductive hormones. GnRH, in turn, is in control of luteinizing hormone (LH) and follicular stimulating hormone (FSH), both of which are vital to ovulation.

Your hormones need to rise and fall at the right levels and the right time like an orchestra playing a complicated sonata. The conductor of this orchestra is GnRH with melatonin in the percussion section helping with the tempo; LH and FSH are important soloists, coming in at just the right time.

Melatonin in implantation

Within a successful reproductive cycle, a good quality egg matures, is released from the ovary during ovulation, fertilizes, and finally, implants into the uterine lining.

Melatonin is important in all of this, including implantation.

Invader alert! Your body needs to suppress the local immune system so that you don't react to the embryo as foreign, and your body also must increase certain proteins that are important for implantation in the uterine wall. Melatonin helps to make both of those activities take place.

How is melatonin made?

Melatonin is secreted mainly by the pineal gland. Serotonin, a neurotransmitter, is converted into melatonin through a couple of steps, one of which includes adding a methyl group. A methyl group is a small molecule made of one carbon surrounded by three hydrogen atoms. This ties back to your need for folate during conception in order to have enough methyl groups.

When light, specifically light in the blue wavelength, hits your eye, it causes a signal to be sent to the brain that suppresses melatonin. Thus, during the day, your body has very low levels of melatonin. At night, melatonin levels begin to rise again around sunset. Your melatonin levels normally peak in the middle of your sleep cycle.

Studies on supplementing with melatonin for fertility

Several recent studies and clinical trials use supplemental melatonin for increasing fertility.

- Women with PCOS who struggled with fertility participated in a six-month trial with supplemental melatonin. The results showed that melatonin regulated the reproductive hormones (FSH, anti-Müllerian, and androgens) and restored the menstrual cycle for many of the women.[2]

- A study of over one hundred women undergoing IVF found that 3 mg of melatonin each night increased fertilization rates by 30%.[3]

- A large IVF trial in women with PCOS found that a combination of melatonin and myo-inositol increased in-vitro fertilization rates.[4]

Supplemental melatonin

Melatonin is available over-the-counter in several forms: tablets, gummies, liquid, fast-melts, and timed-release capsules. Melatonin is quickly absorbed and raises serum levels to a peak within one to two hours of taking it.

The timed-release formulations better mimic natural melatonin levels and sustain the levels over the course of the night so timed-release formulations are recommended.

While most of the trials for fertility used doses of 3 mg/night, people tolerate melatonin supplements differently. Some report side effects of headaches, slight nausea, or grogginess after taking too much melatonin. This may be something that you want to try on a weekend, and you may need to try several different doses to find the right fit for your body.

Supplemental melatonin is available in timed-release capsules ranging from 300 mcg to 5 mg. If you aren't already used to taking melatonin, start with the lower dose 300 mcg and build up to 1 mg or more over the course of a couple of weeks.

Why are everyone's melatonin levels low these days?

Light in the morning is your body's signal to turn off melatonin production. Similarly, light in the blue wavelengths at night also suppress the rise of melatonin levels.

Throughout human history, the only light at night was from the moon and from fire (torches, candles, oil lanterns, etc.). Light from a fire has little to no blue wavelengths, and thus it has no impact on melatonin levels.

Fast forward to our modern era of watching TV while simultaneously surfing smartphones in the evening. Everything with a screen gives off lots of light in the blue wavelengths. To make it worse, the new energy-saving LED light bulbs are also full of light in the blue spectrum.

3 Steps you can take today to boost melatonin:

o   Block out blue light at night. Either turn off electronics (TV, laptops, cell phones, tablets) and dim the overhead lighting two hours before bedtime or wear blue-blocking glasses that block 100% of the blue light for two hours before bedtime.

o   Get some sunlight every morning. Head outside for a walk shortly after the sun comes up. Or drink your coffee on the porch each morning.

o   Consider supplementing with low-dose, timed-release melatonin.

CHAPTER 8

What Should You Eat to Enhance Your Odds of Getting Pregnant?

The proper preconception diet is critical to providing the essential nutrients needed for anyone trying to conceive.

Choosing the right fertility foods to eat when trying to conceive will dramatically increase your chances of getting pregnant. Certain foods good for fertility improve egg quality more than others. These foods help ovulation as well.

What is most important in your preconception diet? In this section, we will discuss the following:

- Getting enough fat and the right type of fat
- Eating good quality protein
- Avoiding the pesticides that zap fertility
- Staying hydrated

Why is your diet so important for fertility?

If you are having a hard time getting pregnant, take a good look at your diet. Yes, there are people who get pregnant while eating junk food and drinking soda, but unsurprisingly, research shows that isn't your best pre-conception diet.

Looking ahead past just getting pregnant, you want your own nutrition to be optimized for giving your baby its best start.

A recent study investigated the diet of couples undergoing IVF treatment. The results showed that a Mediterranean style diet that was high in vegetables, fish, legumes, and olive oil increased the probability of pregnancy by 40%. Women eating the Mediterranean diet had higher folate and vitamin B6 levels.[1]

Another study also on patients at an IVF clinic found that those in the upper half of the healthy diet pattern (fruits, nuts, vegetables, meat, olives, and legumes) were 86% more likely to become pregnant than those in the bottom of the unhealthy pattern, which included junk food and solid oils.[2]

Include enough fat in your diet

Louise's Story

Like most women I had treated, Louise consumed very little fat. She bought non-fat milk and yogurt for breakfast. Her snacks were typically fruit so were fat-free. Although her fat intake was adequate for her needs, I felt that it was short of what was needed for a healthy pregnancy.

I advised her to start including wild salmon, grass-fed butter, and coconut oil in her foods every day. At first she was hesitant about increasing her intake so much, but she eventually got used to the new additions. She realized how much more she enjoyed her foods, even salmon, which she hadn't liked previously.

Her first IVF at age 38 ended with only one embryo to transfer that did not implant. After implementing my *recommended nutritional changes for six months, she did another IVF cycle which resulted in three embryos and a successful pregnancy.*

Eating the right fats is important for a healthy baby.

The brain is made largely of fat (around 60%), and the majority of that fat in the brain is saturated.

The myelin sheath that surrounds the nerves in the brain and ensures their proper function is also largely made of saturated fat and cholesterol.

For that reason, consuming saturated fats is extremely important. This is true both when trying to conceive and during pregnancy.

Eating the right fats is not only important for your future baby but also essential for fertility.

Fats are the basic building blocks of your cell membranes. These fatty membranes surround every cell, including your eggs, and act as the border patrol allowing the right balance of hormones to enter your cells. Healthy cell walls mean a healthy hormone balance. Unhealthy fats make your cell walls rigid, which makes it hard for hormones to get into your cells.

Studies show that low fat diets can decrease ovulation. That's because fats are a structural component for hormones and hormone-like substances. In fact, cholesterol is converted to all hormones, including progesterone, estrogen, testosterone, cortisol, DHEA, and vitamin D.

One study in college-aged women found that those who often skipped their periods ate a diet that contained a lot of omega-6 polyunsaturated fat and little saturated fat.[3]

Fatty fish, such as salmon and albacore tuna, may help to delay menopause. A study in the United Kingdom found that women who included more fish that were high in fat in their diet delayed menopause by 3.3 years per portion of fatty fish eaten each day.[4]

Vegetarian and vegan diets often are low in fat, especially saturated fat. The statistics show that menstrual problems are more common in vegetarians.[5]

Fat soluble vitamins, such as vitamins A, D, E, and K, are best absorbed with fat, so when you eat a low-fat diet, you lose vital fertility nutrients.

Fat provides fuel for mitochondria and produces less damaging free radicals than sugar or carbohydrates.

Saturated or unsaturated fats?

The different types of fats are defined by their chemical structure. Fats are made up mainly of carbon and hydrogen atoms, and the way that they are bonded together defines their structure.

Saturated fats have single bonds between all of the carbons and hydrogens. Because it has the maximum number of hydrogens bonded to the carbons, it's *saturated* with hydrogen atoms. This creates a straight chain and also allows them to pack together more tightly. Saturated fats like butter and coconut oil tend to be solids at room temperature.

Unsaturated fats have at least one carbon-carbon double bond, which causes a bend in the molecule. The bent fatty acids can't pack together as tightly, making them a liquid at room temperature.

Monounsaturated fats (MUFAs) have one carbon-carbon double bond (thus the "mono") with all of the remainder carbon atoms being single-bonded. Examples of foods with high monounsaturated fats are avocados, olive oil, and nuts. They are liquid at room temperature but will become solid when chilled.

Polyunsaturated fats (PUFAs) have two or more carbon-carbon double bonds in their structure. The more double bonds a fat has, the more unstable it becomes to heat. This instability makes it more likely to become rancid, producing damaging free radicals.

What are omega-3 fatty acids?

Omega-3 fatty acids are polyunsaturated fats with several double bonds in the chemical structure.

They have a double bond as their third bond. Omega-3 fats are called *essential* fatty acids because we can't make it on our own and must obtain it through our diet.

Examples of oils that are high in omega-3 fatty acids include:

- Flaxseed
- Chia seed
- Fish oil

Oils that are high in omega-6 fatty acids include soybean, corn, sunflower, cottonseed, walnut, and peanut oil. The ratio of omega-6 to omega-3 fatty acids is important in your diet. Most people today get too much omega-6 and not enough omega-3 fats in their diet.

There are three main omega-3 fatty acids in the diet:

- ALA (alpha-linolenic acid)
- EPA (eicosapentaenoic acid)
- DHA (docosahexaenoic acid)

DHA is the most important omega-3 fatty acid in the human body. It's found in fatty fish, fish oil, grass-fed meat, and pasture-raised eggs.

While your body can convert ALA and EPA to DHA, that conversion is severely limited in some people due to genetic variants. The conversion is also almost non-existent in babies and young children, making DHA an essential part of their diet.

How much DHA do you need?

It is recommended that women who are pregnant or trying to get pregnant consume 300 mg or more of DHA each day.[6]

A study that looked at DHA consumption over the last decade found that over 95% of adults consume less than 250 mg of DHA and EPA combined. So the odds are pretty good that you need to add more DHA to your diet.[7]

DHA for fertility

While DHA is vital for a healthy baby, it is also extremely important when trying to conceive.

An animal study makes clear that supplementing with omega-3s helps with egg quality. The study found that supplementing with omega-3 fatty acids helped to extend the age range for fertility as well as improve the quality of the oocyte.[8]

But what about humans? Studies show that women who have higher intakes of omega-3 fatty acids are more likely to get pregnant than women with the lowest intake.

A study of 501 couples who were trying to conceive clearly shows the importance of DHA in the diet. When both the male and female partners consumed eight or more servings of seafood per month, they had a 61% greater rate of pregnancy and shorter time to conception.[9]

This isn't just for moms-to-be, though. Studies on male infertility show the benefits in sperm motility and sperm count from omega-3 supplements.[10]

For women undergoing in-vitro fertilization, higher levels of DHA are associated with a higher birth rate.[11]

Essential for baby's development

Looking beyond just trying to conceive, higher DHA levels are important for the health of the baby. DHA is incorporated into the neurons of the brain and essential for the baby's development.

Low DHA levels have been linked in several studies to an increased risk of preterm births. A Danish study found that women with the lowest levels of DHA were at a tenfold risk of having their baby prematurely.[12]

A U.S. study found that women who supplemented with 600 mg DHA had babies with greater birth weight and larger head size and were more likely to be full term.[13]

The benefits of DHA go beyond pregnancy. Women who had higher DHA levels while they were pregnant ended up having babies with better problem-solving skills when they were 12 months old.[14]

Plant versus animal sources of DHA

You will often see flaxseed and chia seeds mentioned as good sources of DHA and EPA. These plant sources contain an omega-3 fatty acid called alpha linolenic acid that need to be converted by the body into DHA and EPA. For a portion of the population, this conversion pathway doesn't work well.

The FADS1 gene controls the conversion of omega-3s from plant sources into DHA and EPA. There is a common genetic variant that reduces that conversion for many people. Relying on flaxseed or chia seeds for DHA is not a good idea for people who carry the FADS1 variant.

Adding more DHA into your diet

With 95% of people not consuming enough DHA, these tips for adding more DHA to your pre-pregnancy diet are important for almost everyone.

Eating fish and seafood is an excellent, whole food way to increase your DHA, but women who are trying to conceive need to be careful about too much mercury. The FDA recommends that women who are pregnant or breastfeeding avoid eating swordfish, shark, king mackerel, or tilefish.[15]

The Environmental Working Group has an interactive calculator that gives fish recommendations based on age, gender, and whether you are trying to get pregnant. Their advice includes avoiding orange roughie, sole, flounder, and canned tuna due to mercury contamination. They recommend that women trying to get pregnant include the high omega-3 fish sources, such as salmon, sardines, mackerel, oysters, mussels, rainbow trout, and pollock.[16]

DHA supplements

Another great option is to take a supplement that is high in DHA. There are both fish oil and algal oil (vegetarian) options available. This gives you an easy way to ensure that you are getting enough DHA each day.

How much should you take? Many of the studies on pregnancy and fertility used 600 mg doses of DHA. There is no set RDA for DHA specifically in the U.S.

Fermented cod liver oil is also high in DHA along with vitamin A and D, making it a superior option to most processed fish oil supplements.

What are omega-6 fats?

Another type of polyunsaturated fatty acids, omega-6 fats, are abundant in most people's diet. These fats used to be promoted as being a heart-healthy alternative to saturated fats, but studies now show that omega-6 fats can be pro-inflammatory, possibly contributing to chronic diseases.

Oil	Omega-6	Omega-3
Safflower	75%	0%
Sunflower	65%	0%
Corn	54%	0%
Cottonseed	50%	0%
Soybean	51%	9%

Historically, people consumed a lot less omega-6 fats than they do today. Prior to the industrialization of agriculture and the production of seed oils, people consumed more saturated fat and more omega-3 fats in their diets. Studies show that reducing omega-6 fats back to more historical levels can increase the anti-inflammatory effects of omega-3 fats.[17]

Avoid excess omega-6 fats when trying to conceive

A diet high in omega-6 fats has been directly shown to decrease egg quality. This was due to an increase in oxidative stress within the egg cell.[18]

Where are all these omega-6 fats coming from?

- Fried fast foods are most often cooked in vegetable oil. Usually, vegetable oil is a combination of corn oil, soybean oil, and canola oil—high in omega-6 fatty acids with very little omega-3.

- Another source of omega-6 fats in your diet may be hiding in your salad dressing. Check the label. Soybean oil is often the first ingredient.

- Mayonnaise and other sauces are another big source of omega-6 fats.

- To put it bluntly, if you are serious about trying to conceive, give up fried foods, find a salad dressing that isn't high in omega-6, and start reading ingredient labels.

Protein is vital for fertility

You need protein to build bones, muscles, skin, and cells. Because your body can't store protein the way you can store carbohydrates and fat, you need to get enough protein every day.

When you eat protein, your body digests it and breaks it down into amino acids. Then you can use the amino acids to construct the different proteins that your body and the developing egg cell and embryo need.

The quality of your protein source matters. You don't want your body to have to detoxify a lot of herbicides to get your daily protein.

While beef can be a good source of protein, choosing grass-fed beef improves the quality. The types of fat in the beef are altered in cows that are raised in a feedlot. Grass-fed beef has been shown in several studies to have higher omega-3 fatty acids, which improves the omega-6 to omega-3 ratio.

Free-range chicken is a superior quality protein source when compared to conventionally raised chickens. Cage-free or pasture-raised eggs are also better choices with a naturally higher omega-3 fatty acid content.

Food	Serving Size	Calories	Protein
Chicken	3 oz	141	28 g
Steak	3 oz	158	26 g
Lamb	3 oz	172	23 g
Egg, large	2 eggs	142	12 g
Salmon	3 oz	155	22 g
Chickpeas	½ cup	134	7 g
Quinoa	½ cup	111	4 g

adapted from https://www.todaysdietitian.com/pdf/webinars/Protein ContentofFoods.pdf

If you normally eat a diet that is low in protein, adding more high-quality protein may help you get pregnant. A study of women undergoing IVF found that increasing protein intake and decreasing carbohydrate intake more than tripled their clinical pregnancy rate.[19]

Water

Becky's Story

On her initial visit, Becky noted that she produced very little fertile cervical mucus prior to ovulation for no more than one day. After increasing her water intake dramatically, she reported that she had more cervical mucus the next month, lasting three days. In subsequent cycles, she continued to produce noticeable quantities of the fertile egg-white, stretchy cervical mucus that's optimal for fertilization.

While most people don't think about water when it comes to their diet, it is important to stay hydrated when trying to conceive.

Adequate water intake is essential for healthy egg maturation because without sufficient water, your body can't process nutrients and hormones.

Clinical experience shows that increasing water intake helps increase cervical mucus. This is important because of its role in transporting the sperm to the fallopian tubes for fertilization.

For the fetus, staying hydrated is critical for fetal development. Water helps carry nutrients to the placenta and is an important part of all aspects of development from the time of fertilization. Without water, a developing baby cannot survive, increasing the risk of miscarriage.

Avoid pesticides by eating organic

You go to the grocery store to pick up a couple of apples and some salad fixings. Standing in front of the display of apples, you once again question whether the extra cost for organic apples is worth it.

You may wonder. Is there real research showing that eating organic matters? Will eating organic help you get pregnant? Yes! Research shows that eating conventionally grown fruits and vegetables that contain pesticide residue can reduce your chances of getting pregnant.

Avoiding pesticides by eating organic is important for fertility. Now let's dig into the science to see why this is true.

What does the "organic" label mean?

In the U.S. for a product to be certified as organic, it has to meet standards set by the U.S. Department of Agriculture. These standards include specific farming practices and a focus on sustainability. The organic standards also limit the types of pesticides used. Most of the synthetic pesticides, growth hormones, and synthetic fertilizers are prohibited.

On the other hand, conventional agriculture usually involves using synthetic fertilizers and pesticides when growing crops.

Does organic food contain more nutrients?

The answer may surprise you. Organic and conventionally grown foods are similar in their nutrient profiles.

A few specific foods have higher antioxidant capacity in the organically grown vegetables. Specifically, organic onions have more flavonoids available.

To be fair, a couple of studies show that a few conventionally grown crops, such as oranges, may have a little higher antioxidant capacity.

If organic food isn't wildly more nutritious, why does it affect fertility?

The research shows that the presence of pesticides on conventionally grown foods is reducing fertility for both men and women.[20]

The study participants were 325 women who were undergoing ART (assisted reproductive technology, such as IVF) at Massachusetts General Hospital Fertility Clinic.

Researchers assessed their exposure to pesticides, determining overall fruit and vegetable consumption and how often they chose organic produce.

When the researchers divided the participants by the amount of conventionally grown fruits and vegetables, a significant difference was seen.

The women who consumed a lower amount of pesticide residue (bottom 25%) were 26% more likely to give birth than those who ate more foods with pesticide residue (top 25%).

The women in the low pesticide group ate less than one serving a day of conventionally grown (high pesticide) fruits and vegetables. The women in the high pesticide group were eating more than 2.3 servings per day of conventional fruits and vegetables.

Does eating organic affect sperm quality?

Recent studies have investigated the question of how pesticide residue impacts sperm quality.

One study found that men who ate more servings of fruits and vegetables with pesticide residue had lower sperm counts. When comparing the high pesticide (top 25%) versus low pesticide (bottom 25%) groups, the men who ate more fruit and vegetables with pesticide residue had a 49% lower total sperm count.

Eating organic or avoiding conventionally grown produce makes a big difference for men! The total amount of fruits and vegetables eaten didn't relate to sperm quality; only the amount of pesticide residue was important in this study.[21]

Another study found similar results. Looking at the other side of the picture, the results showed that men who ate higher amounts of organic fruits and vegetables had sperm concentrations that were about 170% higher than that of men who ate less of the organic produce.[22]

Getting specific on pesticides

Not all fruits and vegetables have high amounts of pesticide residue on them. The Environmental Working Group, a nonprofit activist group, comes out with a ranking each year of the fruits and vegetables with the highest burden of pesticide residue.

Their 2019 list of foods with the highest pesticide residue (the *Dirty Dozen*) includes:

- Strawberries
- Spinach
- Kale
- Nectarines
- Apples
- Grapes
- Peaches
- Cherries
- Pears
- Tomatoes
- Celery
- Potatoes

This is an eye-opening list for anyone who makes a morning green smoothie using conventionally grown spinach and kale!

Practical advice on avoiding pesticide residue

If you are trying to get pregnant, both you and your partner should avoid eating conventionally grown fruit and produce with high pesticide content. This means at a minimum you should avoid eating conventionally grown produce on the EWG's *Dirty Dozen* list.

There are fruits and vegetables that don't have as much pesticide residue when conventionally grown. If you have a tight budget for groceries, you can save a little money by sometimes buying conventionally grown produce from the Environmental Working Group's *Clean 15* list.

The EWG's 2019 *Clean 15* list includes:

- Avocado
- Sweet Corn
- Pineapple
- Sweet Peas, Frozen
- Onion
- Papaya
- Eggplant
- Asparagus
- Kiwis
- Cabbage
- Cauliflower
- Cantaloupe
- Broccoli
- Mushroom
- Honeydew Melon

Additionally, you should try to limit your exposure to household pesticides that have been recently sprayed.

Dairy

Dairy is one of the most confusing food groups because so many people rely on drinking milk daily to get their calcium.

Unfortunately, industrial milk and dairy products can be loaded with hormones, antibiotics, and toxins. For example, plastic milk jugs can transfer phthalates into the milk.

Dairy products are a large source of hormones in our diet. Milk includes hormones, such as estrogen, corticosteroids, and testosterone.

While the science isn't entirely clear yet on whether dairy products are harmful when trying to conceive, this may be a time when you want to limit or avoid dairy altogether. Often, dairy is a hidden source of inflammatory reactions for people as well, so eliminating dairy for a period of time can help to calm reactions to it.

If you choose to consume milk products, grass-fed dairy has been shown to have a superior fatty-acid profile as compared to conventionally grown dairy. It has a better omega-6 to omega-3 ratio, and the mix of saturated to unsaturated fats is better. Cows that graze in a pasture all day produce a higher quality milk than cows that are eating industrial farmed grains.

Be sure to get plenty of calcium from other food sources, such as dark, leafy greens, sardines, broccoli, almonds, and sprouted seeds.

.

CHAPTER 9

Leptin: A Hormone that Links Your Weight to Fertility

Researchers have known for years that women who are either overweight or underweight have decreased fertility. But why? This question has been recently answered through research.

Studies that just look at body mass index (BMI) find that women who have a BMI greater than 27 to 29 are at an increased risk for infertility.[1] Similarly, women with a BMI of less than 20 also have lower fertility.[2] Of course, studies vary on the exact BMI levels, and some of it depends on ethnic background. For example, women of East Asian background may not be at an increased risk of infertility unless they are at a BMI less than 18.5.[3]

When you zoom out and look at reproduction from a higher level, it's obvious that pregnancy should only take place when conditions are right. But reproduction is an energy-intensive process, especially for mammals.

One fundamental factor for getting pregnant is to have enough fuel available. Not enough food means either baby or mom won't be healthy. Therefore, your body knows that the conditions aren't right for pregnancy.

ENOUGH NUTRIENTS = OKAY TO HAVE BABY.

The key here is that your body produces a signaling molecule which tells your brain there is enough fuel. It's kind of like a gas gauge on a car. You wouldn't start out on a long road trip with no gas, and your body doesn't want to start down the reproductive path without enough fuel.

The same signaling molecule is also involved in telling your body both that there is enough fuel (stop eating) and that it is time to be fertile.

That signaling hormone is called leptin. Research studies on leptin explain why it is an integral part of fertility. The studies show exactly how it signals that the time is right for reproducing.[4]

Leptin: a hormone controlling both appetite and fertility

Leptin is a hormone secreted by your adipose (fat) tissue. When leptin levels are low, it triggers your drive to eat more. When you have plenty of fat tissue, leptin levels are high, decreasing your appetite.

In 1994, a geneticist named Jeffrey Friedman first discovered the gene that produces leptin. This hormone quickly became known as a major player in obesity. For people who don't produce enough leptin, the signal that the body has enough stored fuel doesn't reach the brain.

People with a rare mutation that drastically reduces their leptin are always hungry and quickly become obese. The low leptin levels tell their brain that they are starving. They are driven to eat more, starting as an infant, but there is another sign of leptin deficiency that puzzled scientists for a long time. Leptin deficiency also causes delayed puberty and infertility.[5]

Leptin is more than just a hunger hormone. It also signals to the reproductive systems that all is well and ready for baby.

How does leptin influence reproductive hormones?

In the brain, there is a small region called the hypothalamus. It is only about the size of an almond, but it controls a lot of important functions in your body. The hypothalamus controls your body temperature, appetites, circadian rhythm, sleep, and most importantly, the regulation of reproductive hormones.

Within the hypothalamus, different groups of neurons perform different functions. One of these groups of neurons controls signaling for reproductive hormones, and leptin is a trigger for these neurons.

Gonadotropin-releasing hormone (GnRH) is controlled by the hypothalamus. GnRH is responsible for signaling the pituitary to release the follicle-stimulating hormone (FSH) and luteinizing hormone (LH).

FSH and LH are the hormones that control the creation of the egg and ovulation. You have to have FSH and LH in the right amounts and at the right time for menstruation or pregnancy.

This pathway of signaling for the reproductive hormones is called the hypothalamic-pituitary-gonadal (HPG) axis.[6]

As one study states, "Serum leptin levels are a critical link between sufficient nutrition and the function of the hypothalamic–pituitary–gonadal (HPG) axis."

Specific neurons in the hypothalamus receive the leptin signal and are responsible for both the normal onset of puberty and normal fertility. More importantly, this signaling action is completely independent of the way that leptin controls appetite and metabolism.

Low leptin levels (and low BMI) can cause infertility.

Low leptin levels signal that there isn't enough food available and thus we shouldn't reproduce.

Animal studies have shown this repeatedly.

Research backs this up in an easy-to-grasp experiment. A double-blind placebo-controlled trial of prescription leptin was conducted on lean women (BMI <20) who no longer had their periods. Giving them a prescription leptin medication restored menstruation for 70% of the women. They didn't have to gain weight or eat more. They just needed the signal that tells the brain to release the reproductive hormones.[7]

Intense exercise

Women who exercise excessively or who are competitive athletes will often find that they stop having their periods. This is due to low leptin levels, which cause low levels of hypothalamic stimulation of gonadal hormones. The medical term for this is hypothalamic amenorrhea.

Women who are involved in leanness sports (e.g., runners, gymnasts, bikers, dancers, and swimmers) may not produce enough leptin. In fact, a study of women athletes participating in college sports found that almost 25% of women competing in leanness sports had menstrual dysfunctions.[8]

This is a known problem and not limited to elite athletes. Studies show that chronic energy deficiency due to overexercising and undereating is the cause of not ovulating for about 30% of women. Restoring leptin levels in these women will cause them to regain normal menstrual cycles, allowing them to become pregnant.

Leptin resistance and infertility

Kendra's Story

At 39 years, Kendra was severely overweight and had been for years. She had tried many diets to no avail and had given up on losing weight. Her three insemination cycles with Clomid and one IVF were all unsuccessful. She was open to trying anything, so I immediately changed her nutrition and got her to start walking three times a week. Over the next twelve months, she lost almost 40 pounds. She was still overweight, but she lost enough weight for her to get pregnant.

But wait, what about women who are overweight? Researchers find that almost all people who are overweight have higher leptin levels, so it isn't a lack of leptin, but rather a lack of receiving the hormone's signal that is playing a role in overeating. The fat cells are producing plenty of leptin, but that signal isn't reaching the brain correctly.

The fact that overweight people have higher leptin levels has led scientists to conclude that the signal from leptin is not getting through to the hypothalamus. This is termed *leptin resistance*.

The inability to receive the leptin signal can also impair fertility.

Studies of women with unexplained infertility find decreased leptin receptor function and higher than normal leptin levels in the follicular fluid. Additionally, leptin in the ovarian follicles needs to be at the right amount. Too high of leptin levels in the follicles is linked to decreased fertility.

Researchers think that leptin resistance is one of the causes of being overweight/obese.

The leptin signal is not being received in the brain, and thus the control system for weight is out of balance.

85

This same leptin resistance that causes people to gain weight may be causing problems when trying to conceive. If the hypothalamus isn't receiving the leptin signal, your body may decrease reproductive hormones.

There are several theories why people have leptin resistance.

- One theory is that when leptin levels are too high in the bloodstream, it decreases the amount that can cross the blood brain barrier into the brain. The signal doesn't reach the hypothalamus.

- Another possibility is that low-grade, chronic inflammation in the hypothalamus decreases the leptin receptor function.

Putting all of the research together shows that:

- Low amounts of leptin—either through lack of food or leptin deficiency—impairs fertility. This is a problem for women who have very low body fat.

- More often, though, women have a problem with higher weight. Almost all overweight women are producing high amounts of leptin, but that signal isn't being received correctly in the brain. The brain is resistant to the leptin hormone signal.

- Leptin hormone resistance causes at least two issues: increased appetite and altered reproductive hormones.

- The increased appetite/weight and decreased fertility are two separate conditions. Fertility is impaired through changes in the hypothalamus-pituitary-gonadal (HPG) axis and subsequent changes to LH and FSH levels.

- Whether through lack of leptin hormone or leptin resistance, the impact on reproductive hormone signaling results in decreased fertility.

What can you do if you suspect that leptin resistance is sabotaging your ability to get pregnant?

In general, leptin sensitivity is a balancing act between the signal getting to your brain and the brain receiving the signal.

Sleep is absolutely vital for leptin sensitivity. Leptin levels are not only controlled by your body fat and eating, but they vary according to your circadian rhythm. Melatonin has recently been shown to be important in the production and regulation of leptin. An animal study found that removing the melatonin receptor caused leptin resistance. Adding in extra melatonin reversed the leptin problems and restored fertility to the animals.[10]

Not getting enough sleep affects both leptin levels and BMI. The amount of time spent in REM sleep is also associated with leptin levels.

A recent study showed that bright light in the morning can also help to restore leptin levels, especially when sleep deprived. The study used full spectrum light, so getting outside in the morning sunshine is a great way to get your bright light.[11]

If you are overweight

For anyone who is overweight, decreasing fat mass—i.e., losing weight—is the sure-fire way to lower leptin levels.

Weight loss needs to be done carefully when you are trying to conceive. This is not a time to go on a crash diet or use unregulated diet pills.

Sticking to a diet that is high in whole foods, such as vegetables and meats, while eliminating processed foods is a great way to maintain your nutrient balance while losing some weight. Getting regular, moderate exercise is important, but this is also not the time to go overboard by exercising too much.

High fructose consumption has been linked to leptin resistance, so eliminating high fructose corn syrup from your diet is a must.

High triglyceride levels have been linked in several studies to leptin resistance. Excessive carbohydrate consumption is one cause of high triglycerides, so eating a lower or more moderate amount of carbohydrates can help to lower your triglycerides. High fructose consumption also elevates triglyceride levels for some people, so avoid foods with added fructose.

Finally, a protein in wheat and legumes can bind to the leptin receptor, blocking it from receiving the leptin signal. While this may not be a big component of leptin resistance, trying a wheat and legume-free diet is a good idea. Instead of breads and pasta, substitute extra servings of organic vegetables. Instead of legumes, eat more wild fatty fish like salmon.

Solutions for a low BMI

If you have been constantly dieting for years, it is time to take stock of your eating habits and calculate your BMI using an online calculator.

If your BMI is below 19, it is a good indication that gaining a little weight may raise your leptin levels.

If you are unsure whether low leptin is the problem, you can get a simple, inexpensive blood test done to check your leptin levels. Leptin levels are highest in the morning, so you may want to get the blood test done in the afternoon for a true measure of your status.

A healthy diet that includes enough fat from fish, grass-fed beef, and pasture raised eggs may be all that you need to increase your leptin levels.

If you exercise a lot or are training as an athlete, cutting back on exercise to a more moderate amount may restore your leptin levels and your fertility.

5 steps you can take today to increase your sensitivity to leptin:

- o   Reduce your triglyceride levels if they are high. Lowering your carbohydrates and specifically avoiding high fructose corn syrup may help to lower triglycerides.

- o   If you are overweight, try losing weight through a nutrient dense diet that includes organic meats and vegetables.

- o   Exercise in moderation.

- o   Sleep well and avoid blue light for two hours before bed.

- o   Eliminate wheat and legumes from your diet.

CHAPTER 10

Lifestyle Changes that Promote Fertility

This is the time to put all your effort into optimizing diet and lifestyle for fertility. But you don't have to drive yourself nuts when doing so!

Here are some tips for improving your lifestyle and the science that backs up the suggestions.

Knowing the research will help you to understand why these changes are important so you can determine what is best for *you*.

Exercise, but don't overexercise

We all know that exercise is important. It is good for your overall health, and studies show that exercise improves your ability to get pregnant.

BUT too much exercise will stress out your body and reduce fertility chances.

There are often two extremes when it comes to people and exercise–those who overdo it and those who don't do it at all! *You know which camp you fall into.*

This section is divided into two parts:

- Motivation and scientific facts for the couch potatoes (or people who are too busy and too tired to exercise)
- Reality check and studies for the five-day a week spin-class guru

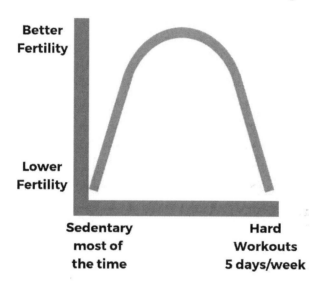

Exercise and Fertility

Better Fertility

Lower Fertility

Sedentary most of the time

Hard Workouts 5 days/week

Studies on how exercise affects fertility

For the couch potato

What does your typical day look like? For a lot of women, it involves getting up and heading to work each day. Let me explain that in terms of activity level. Grab a cup of coffee and head out the door to sit in your car for 40 minutes in traffic. Head into the office to sit at a desk for four or five hours each morning. Walk down to the nearby restaurant and sit and chat with co-workers for lunch. Back to the office where you buckle down and sit for four more hours in the afternoon. Out the door to your car where you sit for 40 minutes (unless there is an accident, and that makes it 50 minutes) on the way home from work. Fix dinner and then sit and watch Netflix for a couple of hours.

Did that perfectly describe your normal workday?

You may have a great, interesting, or exciting job. But the simple fact is that your body is not designed to sit for the majority of the day.

How bad is it to be sedentary? Does this really affect your fertility?

It may surprise you to know that sedentary behavior–sitting at a desk most of the day–was shown in a study to increase the risk of infertility by 260%.[1]

It is time to get moving! While you may not be a couch potato per se, office jobs that entail a lot of sitting can negatively impact your fertility.

3 Steps you can take today to get more active:

o   Get up and move around for a few minutes every hour. If you have an activity monitor, like a Fitbit or Oura ring, set it so that it reminds you hourly to move if you haven't. Otherwise, set a reminder on your cell phone. Get up and walk around the office, do some air squats, take a dance break–just move!

o   Take a brisk walk after lunch. Get others in your office involved as well to increase your accountability.

o   Get in the habit of parking farther away from stores and the office. You will get more exercise, and you will

> *leave those front parking spots available for an elderly person who needs it.*

For the five-day a week spin class guru

Hannah's Story

Hannah's stink eye told me exactly what she thought about my recommendation to cut down on her workout routine. At 43 years old, she was in enviably fit shape with lean, defined muscles. Her body fat percentage was too low, though. So low that it affected her menstrual cycle – coming sporadically. Because of its unpredictability, she could never figure out when she was ovulating. Much to her consternation, I advised her to reduce her daily, intensive 1.5 hour exercise regimen to a more reasonable four to five times a week frequency, lasting no longer than one hour with each session. VERY reluctantly, she decreased her hours in the gym. She stuck it out for the year that it took for her to get pregnant with her baby girl.

It is time to give your body a break!

Overexercising is a known factor for stopping ovulation. The syndrome known as the female athlete triad is defined as female athletes who no longer have periods and have low bone mineral density. This affects both high level athletes as well as women who train hard and often without allowing time for recovery and without eating enough calories.

Moderate exercise is important, but the key word there is *moderate*. Balance is essential here.

If you have stopped having your period due to overexercising, it is often because your body knows that there isn't enough energy available for reproduction. In a study of elite athletes who no longer had periods, adding 360 more calories of carbohydrate plus protein was enough to bring back menstruation for most of the study participants.[2]

How much is too much? There is no one-size-fits-all answer. What is too much for one woman may still be okay for another. One study found that over five hours per week of vigorous exercise increased the risk of infertility.[3]

If you work out a lot and have a low BMI, it may be time to take a good look at your diet to make sure you are getting enough nutrients. One study found that it was especially hard for women athletes on a vegetarian or gluten-free diet to get enough energy in their diet to match the expenditure from hard workouts.[4]

Being sedentary most of the day and then working out moderately for an hour at the gym isn't the best solution either. If you sit a lot at work, make time each hour to get up and move around. Look into a standing desk or exercise ball to replace your chair.

Detoxifying your house

Previous chapters explained how chemicals, such as phthalates, BPA, and pesticides, are impacting egg quality. Now for some practical advice on getting your home into shape for your best fertility chances.

Keep in mind: This doesn't have to be expensive, and it doesn't have to happen overnight. These are steps that may take a little time to implement.

Dusting Your Home

Surprisingly, one of the biggest sources of phthalates is in household dust.[5]

You don't need chemicals or sprays for dusting, just use a damp rag. If you need more cleaning power, try a little vinegar and water in a spray bottle.

Don't forget about baseboards and fan blades!

Vacuuming up the toxicants

Similar to dusting, if you have carpeted floors, give them a good cleaning. Again, there is no need for added cleaning products.

If you don't have a HEPA filter on your vacuum, try using a dust mask when you clean.

Containers for your kitchen

You know that microwaving or heating foods in plastic is a problem. It is time to invest in some glass storage containers.

If you don't want to spend the money right now on glass storage containers, at the very least, get in the habit of never heating food in plastic. If you are heating something in the microwave, transfer it to a plate that's not made of plastic. Never use plastic wrap in the microwave to cover food.

Save a few jars for storing things in the fridge. Wide mouth pickle jars are great. Just soak them in hot water to remove the labels.

Laundry detergent and dryer sheets

Simply switching to the *free and clear* laundry detergent options will decrease your exposure to the phthalates used in fragrances.

A major source of phthalates in the body comes from contact with clothes. Cotton has been shown to adsorb phthalates and other chemicals from the air. Washing cotton clothing more often using natural laundry detergent may help to decrease your toxic burden.[6]

Lowering your stress levels

When you've been trying for months or years to get pregnant, stress seems unavoidable. The longer it has been, the more stressed out you might get because time is getting shorter.

However, understanding how stress can affect fertility allows you to proactively manage its effects.

Say you see a tiger crouching in the brush next to the trail, or you nearly get sideswiped in rush hour traffic. Both situations cause your body to activate your two stress response systems by releasing adrenaline and cortisol from your adrenal glands.

You will immediately produce norepinephrine (adrenaline) and get a rush of energy that lets you run from that tiger. Your body will also produce more cortisol which will help your body deal with the stressor by increasing blood glucose levels for quick energy, increasing blood pressure, and decreasing immune response.

This is exactly what you need when there is a tiger chasing you. On the other hand, chronic stress creates all sorts of problems.

Chronic stress comes from driving daily in rush hour traffic, trying to balance a marriage and home life with a career, and dealing with emotional turmoil. Chronic stress can also be due to a physical illness, lingering viruses, exposure to toxins, or eating foods you are slightly allergic to.

Christine's Story

At 38 years, Christine had already experienced the trauma of three consecutive miscarriages. She dreamed of becoming a mother but was terrified of conceiving again and the possibility of another failed pregnancy.

I advised her not to get pregnant immediately but to practice the strategies I taught her to manage her fears. She was under too much stress for a pregnancy to hold.

After a few months of diligently practicing emotional well-being, she was ready to try again, and her resulting pregnancy went to term with a healthy baby.

The problem with chronic stress is that it raises cortisol levels all the time. Your body has a natural rhythm that controls cortisol production at different times of the day. Constantly elevated cortisol levels can cause depression, weight gain, and elevated blood pressure. It also can interfere with trying to conceive.

How your body makes cortisol

The stress response starts in the brain—in the hypothalamus. This area of the brain starts the signaling process to create cortisol.

The hypothalamus produces a signaling molecule called corticotrophin-releasing hormone (CRH). CRH then travels to the pituitary gland, located near the middle of your brain. This causes the pituitary to produce adrenocorticotropic hormone (ACTH). From the pituitary, ACTH travels to the adrenal glands which sit on top of the kidneys, signaling for the production of cortisol.

This whole process of producing cortisol is actually a feedback loop. High cortisol levels signal to the hypothalamus to stop the production of CRH.

When does your body make cortisol?

Normally, your body produces cortisol rhythmically throughout the day and night. This base level of cortisol helps to regulate:

- Body temperature
- Digestion
- Blood glucose levels
- Immune function
- Mood
- Energy

Cortisol helps to keep your body in homeostasis—everything in balance. Without the right amount of cortisol, things can get out of balance.

Your body has two types of cortisol receptors:

- Cortisol binds to mineralocorticoid receptors (MRs) when the levels are low and normal

- Glucocorticoid receptors (GRs) are activated when there is high cortisol, in times of stress

When cortisol binds to the glucocorticoid receptors, it suppresses the inflammatory system, influences memory, changes blood glucose levels, and increases heart function. Again, this is what is supposed to happen when you have been chased by a lion. But you can see that long-term elevation of cortisol can cause problems.

HPA axis dysfunction

When the cortisol response is out of balance —either chronically high or chronically low —it can result in what is known as hypothalamus-pituitary-adrenal (HPA) axis dysfunction.

HPA axis dysfunction can cause:

- Tiredness along with difficulty sleeping

- Stress and feelings of being overwhelmed

- Difficulty concentrating

- Menstrual irregularities

- Weight changes

- Blood sugar regulation problems

- Depression

Your body needs cortisol in the right amount and at the right time.

HPA axis dysfunction can be due to the glucocorticoid receptors not functioning as they should. Altered cortisol rhythms also cause HPA axis dysfunction.

Women naturally have a higher cortisol response to stress than men do. This is due, in part, to men having higher androgen hormone levels. The androgens, such as testosterone, decrease ACTH levels while estrogen increases ACTH.

This may be why some of the chronic stress disorders, such as depression, anxiety, and PTSD, are more common in women than in men. Depressed women have both reduced glucocorticoid receptor function and altered cortisol rhythms.

Infertility and HPA axis dysfunction

It intuitively makes sense that a time of high stress would be the wrong time to reproduce.

Many studies have shown that chronic activation of the HPA axis inhibits fertility. ACTH, the hormone that tells the adrenals to produce cortisol, also causes the adrenals to produce some of the androgen hormones. This changes the balance of certain hormones that are important when trying to get pregnant. It causes a change in the ratio of follicle stimulating hormone to luteinizing hormone (FSH: to LH), which impact egg quality. Chronic stress activation can eventually inhibit estrogen secretion.

Not only can high cortisol levels prevent you from getting pregnant, it also is linked to a significantly increased risk of early term miscarriage.[7]

Stress, whether physical or mental, can thus cause the perfect storm for fertility challenges. Not only does the initial stress cause physical changes in your body, but each month that you don't get pregnant that mental and physical stress ramps up.

Lowering your cortisol levels with lifestyle changes

The first place to start for lowering your cortisol levels is sleep. Cortisol follows your body's circadian rhythm, so keeping that on track with a good sleep routine is important. Try to go to bed at a consistent time each night.

In addition to consistent sleep timing, getting enough sleep each night is important. A study showed that restricting sleep to four hours per night raised cortisol levels the next day by 21%.[8]

When trying to get pregnant, get at least eight to nine hours of sleep each night. Your goal is to wake up refreshed and ready for the day.

Studies show that both yoga and meditation decrease cortisol levels.[9][10]

Chewing during stressful conditions decreases the cortisol stress reaction, so try chewing gum sweetened with xylitol the next time you are going into a stressful confrontation.[11] Doing so will also reduce the need for a smoke or drink as a coping mechanism.

Get outside. Forest bathing, popular in Japan, reduces cortisol levels. While a forest may not be at your back door, you can go for a walk in a local park or on the weekends, hike in a nearby natural area.[12]

Lowering your cortisol with herbs or supplements

Studies show that certain herbs help with HPA axis dysfunction by moderating cortisol response levels. Some commonly used herbs include Ashwagandha and Rhodiola.[13]

Holy Basil, taken either as a supplement or as Tulsi tea, has been shown in studies to inhibit the release of cortisol.[14]

4 Important Lifestyle changes you can start today:

o Get rid of toxicants. Read the ingredients on your personal care products to see if they contain phthalates or parabens. Toss the products that you don't really need, like lotions you received as a holiday gift. Then find healthier alternatives for what you use on a daily basis.

o Start an exercise routine. Often it is easier to stick to a moderate exercise routine if you involve a friend for accountability, so make today the day that you recruit a friend for a daily hour-long walk. First thing in the morning is great for the early day sunlight exposure, but walking with a co-worker may be more convenient. An after-dinner walk with your partner is an excellent way to reconnect after a long day.

o Take a realistic look at what is causing you stress. Is it your job? Relationship with family or friends? Does your daily commute start your day with a lot of stress? Decide on one step you can take today to decrease your stress. If it is a relationship, perhaps backing off on communicating with that person (mute them on Facebook, stop following on Instagram) is needed at this time in your life.

o Nature is a powerful way to reduce stress, and one that we often don't think about in our busy lives. Schedule some down time this week and go for a short hike in a nearby forest. Live in the heart of a big city? Spend some time in a park, botanical garden, or greenway.

Supplements for Enhancing Fertility

The idea that you can get all your nutrients from food is fine, in theory, but virtually impossible in practice. This is especially true if you are trying to achieve a specific health goal like getting pregnant with a healthy baby after years of trying.

As much as we want to eat the right foods 100% of the time, it's not realistic. Busy schedules, vacations, and temptations all work against us. It is often hard to find the time to shop and cook from scratch every day.

Supplements help to bridge the nutritional gap that processed foods create from eating convenient foods with very little nutrients.

Supplements are the ultimate hack. They are shortcuts to get your body functioning optimally. They're concentrated so they help to shorten the time to your end goal of getting pregnant.

Some of the reasons why we can't rely on food alone to get our nutrients are:

- Soil depletion: Our soils are depleted of nutrients from improper farming practices. On top of that, most plants are not harvested fresh. They sit on trucks, shelves, and counters for weeks before being eaten. Over time, the nutrient content of these plants decreases.

- Mineral depletion from our water: Water filtration is essential in removing toxins, but the process strips the water of important minerals.

- Food and environmental toxins: Your body needs nutrients to deal with toxins. The more toxins you're exposed to, the more need for nutrients.

- Poor absorption: As you age, hydrochloric acid and digestive enzyme production naturally decline, making it difficult for you to break down and absorb nutrients from your foods. That's one reason why heartburn and acid reflux become more of a problem. As you get older, you also often begin taking medications which can interfere with nutrient absorption. This means you need to compensate with more nutrients in the most absorbable form possible.

- Prescription and over-the-counter (OTC) medications: The long-term use of prescription and OTC drugs can cause nutrient deficiencies vital to fertility. These include birth control pills, metformin, heartburn medications, aspirin, anti-depressants, medications for heartburn, high blood pressure, high cholesterol, and asthma.[1]

- Stress: Eating behavior is often affected by stress resulting in more frequent snacking and choosing poor quality food to offer comfort.

- Optimal function: This is the most important reason for supplementing when trying to get pregnant. If your body has low nutrient levels, this might manifest with low energy, poor willpower, decreased mental clarity and focus, and, of course, not getting pregnant. Your body has to direct its nutrient reserves to critical, life-giving functions first–digestion, breathing, movement, and thinking. It doesn't have the extra reserves for activities that aren't life-threatening, like getting pregnant. In times of perceived famine, your body will stop reproducing. It thinks there's not enough food for both you and a baby. Obviously, we don't live in times of famine. But we often make poor food choices by eating convenient, processed, pre-packaged foods that have few nutrients; your brain then perceives that you don't have enough nutrients to support another life.

Arianna's Story

Thinking that her diet was enough to supply all the nutrients she needed, Arianna bristled at my list of recommended supplements. She HATED taking pills. I explained to her at 40 years old, the supplements would help to optimize her fertility by improving her egg quality, giving her best chance. Although she was reluctant at first, she credited her pregnancy ten months later to her supplement regimen.

If the nutrient deficiencies go on long enough, they can cause DNA damage and make you age faster, resulting in poor egg quality.

The next sections will go into detail on nutrients that are essential for fertility, explaining the best forms to use and the research that backs up these recommendations.

Folate and vitamin B12 are vital for fertility

What is vitamin B12?

Vitamin B12 is a water-soluble vitamin that is essential for your health. It is also known as cobalamin, which refers to its structure with a cobalt ion at the core.

Your body uses vitamin B12 in methylation cycle reactions. These methylation reactions turn on and off genes, convert serotonin to melatonin, change homocysteine to methionine, and more.

Vitamin B12 is also used in the mitochondria, those powerhouses of the cell, converting fatty acids into energy.

Vitamin B12 deficiency

Meats and dairy products are your dietary sources of B12, so a deficiency can be a real problem if you are eating a vegetarian or vegan diet. Even if you are eating some animal product, medications, such as heartburn remedies, can disrupt your absorption of B12.

The symptoms of severe vitamin B12 deficiency include:

- Memory issues
- Mood swings
- Disorientation
- Numbness
- Appetite loss
- Constipation
- Sore tongue

Vitamin B12 deficiency is also a cause of megaloblastic anemia.

What is vitamin B9 (folate)?

Folate, or vitamin B9, is a general term that refers to both naturally occurring folates in foods as well as synthetic folic acid.

Synthetic folic acid is often added to foods, such as flour, cornmeal, rice, and pasta. The structure of folic acid is a little different from naturally found folates. Folic acid is more chemically stable and cheaper, so it can easily be added to processed foods and supplements.

Your body must convert either folic acid or natural folate into the active form called 5-methyltetrahydrofolate. The body uses folate in the methylation cycle as well.

The U.S. recommended daily allowance (RDA) for pregnancy is 600 mcg/day. Foods high in folate include liver and dark, leafy green vegetables, such as spinach, Brussels sprouts, broccoli, mustard greens, and asparagus.

Folate deficiency

Not getting enough folate in your diet can lead to a higher rate of neural tube defects as well as other birth defects. This prompted the U.S. government to mandate folic acid fortification in wheat and rice products in 1998.

Folate and B12: together and in the right amounts

Both folate and B12 are active within the methylation cycle, which is foundational to so many biological processes.

Researchers have shown that both vitamins are essential in healthy pregnancies.

Over 62% of pregnant women are deficient in vitamin B12. The rates are even higher for vegans and long-term vegetarians.[2]

Studies on folate and B12 show:

- One study investigated the role that folate plays in pregnancy. The study looked at women undergoing IVF, dividing the participants into three groups (low, medium, and high) based on folate levels. The women with high folate levels had more than double the likelihood of pregnancy.[3]

- Another study noted that women referred for IVF were very likely to have inadequate B12 and folate levels. In fact, only 44% of the women had adequate B12 levels, and only 12% had optimal folate levels.[4]

- When looking at embryo quality in IVF, researchers find that higher B12 correlates with healthier embryos. They also find that increased folate in follicles significantly increases the chance of pregnancy.[5]

- This isn't just important for moms-to-be. Dads need vitamin B12, too. A study showed that the amount of B12 in semen correlates to sperm concentration, which is important when trying to conceive.[6] Folate is also very important for sperm motility. Men who are taking acid-suppressing medications are at a higher risk for folate deficiency and infertility.[7]

Avoid excess folic acid

While having enough folate is vital for a healthy pregnancy, too much folic acid may be detrimental. Your body metabolizes, or breaks down, synthetic folic acid differently than folates from food sources. This can lead to unmetabolized folic acid in the bloodstream.

Researchers are still studying the impact of unmetabolized folic acid. Some studies have linked excess folic acid in mothers to an increased risk of autism spectrum disorder in their children. Other studies, though, also point to the importance of having enough folate; low folate is also linked to an increased risk of autism.[8] [9] So if too much folic acid may cause problems, you may be wondering if the same is true of folate from foods, such as leafy green veggies. This doesn't seem to be the case.

Synthetic folic acid is a different chemical compound than folate found naturally in foods. It is metabolized in the liver rather than the intestines. Natural folates from foods are broken down in the intestines, so your body absorbs just the right amount.[10]

The FDA has set the safe upper limit for folic acid at 1,000 mcg/day. If you are taking a prenatal supplement with 800 mcg plus eating fortified foods, such as bread, cereal, pasta, or rice, you may exceed that limit.

Switching to a prenatal supplement with methylfolate helps you to avoid too much folic acid.

While excess unmetabolized folic acid may be a risk factor in pregnancy, one recent animal study showed that adding vitamin B12 can reduce some of the effects.[11]

Vitamin D is important when trying to get pregnant

Adequate levels of vitamin D during pre-conception are required to ensure a healthy pregnancy.

One of its most important roles in fertility is during the implantation process, when it protects the embryo so that the mother's body doesn't attack what is essentially a foreign body. This is proven by the high concentrations of vitamin D in the uterine lining during the first trimester.

A study using egg donors further showed vitamin D's influence on the uterine lining. The results were a 31% live birth rate in vitamin D deficient recipients, compared with 59% among vitamin D sufficient recipients.[12]

What is known about vitamin D's importance to fertility includes its impact on:

- AMH - Vitamin D stimulates anti-Müllerian hormone (AMH) production, which is a measure of ovarian reserve. Vitamin D deficiency is associated with lower ovarian reserve.

- PCOS - Vitamin D supplementation improves insulin resistance and the effects of infertility treatment. Obesity, vitamin D storage in fat tissue, and sun avoidance results in 65% to 87% rate of vitamin D deficiency in PCOS patients.

- Uterine fibroids - A common cause of infertility, fibroids appear more frequently in women with vitamin D deficiency. African Americans are two to three times more likely to have fibroids than Caucasians, correlating with the observation that the average vitamin D levels are lower by almost 50% in African Americans as compared to Caucasians.

- Sperm quality - Low sperm count, motility, and morphology have been linked to low vitamin D levels.

- IVF - In one study, women with high initial vitamin D levels had a four-time better chance for successful IVF procedure compared to the group with low levels.[13]

What is the best source of vitamin D?

This is a simple question to answer. *Sunlight!*

We are solar-powered beings and require the sun for many of our biological functions. However, being indoors for the vast majority of the day contributes to the epidemic of vitamin D insufficiency found in the majority of Americans.

Because 80% of the vitamin D your body makes is from sunlight and the remaining 20% comes from diet and supplements, the best way to increase vitamin D levels is to be in the sun.

Spend 15 to 30 minutes daily, or about half the time it takes your skin to turn pink, in direct sunlight with *no* sunscreen.

109

The goal is to get adequate sun and not burn. Peak times are between 10 a.m. to 3 p.m.

For light skinned people this may be only 15 to 30 minutes, but darker skinned people may need two hours or more in the winter.

Best natural food sources of vitamin D

Vitamin D exists in two forms: vitamin D2 (calciferol or ergocalciferol) and D3 (cholecalciferol).

In animals, ultraviolet B radiation (UVB) converts cholesterol in the skin to D3—thus the root "chole" in its scientific name, cholecalciferol.

D2 is made in fungi (notably mushrooms) and yeast.

Vitamin D intake from foods is of minor significance compared to the sun because very few foods contain vitamin D naturally.

Although getting enough vitamin D from natural food sources alone is difficult, below are some of the best:

- Fatty fish, like wild salmon, mackerel, sardines, herring, wild cod

- Pasture-raised eggs

- Grass-fed beef liver

Farmed fish and conventionally raised chicken and cows are fed genetically modified (GMO) corn and soybeans so they do not develop sufficient levels of vitamin D.

Vegetarian food source of vitamin D

The only vegetarian source of natural vitamin D is mushrooms; however, this form is not the same as that found in animal sources (vitamin D3).

In fact, vitamin D2 is not made in the human body at all and is less effective than the D3 form that we make ourselves. No surprise there.

One study shows that vitamin D3:

- Is 87% better at raising and maintaining vitamin D levels
- Produces two to three times more storage of the vitamin than D2[14]

Therefore, mushrooms should *not* be relied on as a natural food source of vitamin D.

Fortified food sources of vitamin D

Most Americans get the majority of their vitamin D from fortified foods, like milk, cereals, orange juice, and yogurt.

However, your body does not use vitamin D added to foods the same way as getting it from the sun or from foods that naturally contain vitamin D. This is because when you absorb the sun or eat real food, the synergistic effect of other vitamins, minerals, co-factors, and enzymes in that food allow for optimal use by the body.

Without these complementary compounds, synthetic nutrients aren't used in the same way as their natural forms.

Furthermore, fortified foods are processed foods.

The focus of any fertility-enhancing diet is to eat more naturally nutrient-rich whole foods.

How CoQ10 improves egg quality

Mitochondria are the power plants of the cell, including eggs and sperm.

They provide energy by converting food into ATP which fuels the cell's activities.

As we age, the mitochondria become less efficient, and fewer new, healthy ones are made.

Eggs have about 200 times more mitochondria than any other cell. When eggs are developing, they use a tremendous amount of energy.

Early embryo division and implantation also require a lot of energy.

Studies show that the mitochondria of older eggs produce significantly less ATP.

In fact, young egg cells have about 75% more ATP than egg cells from older women.[15] This has a significant impact on fertility as the rate of division and successful implantation of embryos has more to do with how much energy the egg has than with your actual chronological age.[16]

Mitochondrial energy production

Within the mitochondria, 95% of all cellular energy production depends on CoQ10.

CoQ10 is your only fat-soluble antioxidant. As an antioxidant, it protects the eggs from damage caused by toxins.

CoQ10 is also called ubiquinone because it is ubiquitous in the body and is so important that it is made by all of your cells.

Deficiency of CoQ10 is thought to contribute to the accelerated egg loss and poor pregnancy outcomes seen with aging.

However, studies show that supplementing with CoQ10 can be helpful for couples dealing with infertility.

- A study of women undergoing IVF found that CoQ10 increased the number of high-quality eggs.[17]

- Not only for women, CoQ10 supplementation helps sperm quality.[18]

- Animal studies show that CoQ10 specifically increases mitochondrial function in the eggs.[19]

Food sources of CoQ10

Although many people think of CoQ10 as a supplement, you can also get CoQ10 from food.

Unfortunately, most people aren't able to get a significant amount through diet alone. This is because the foods that are highest in CoQ10 are not usually part of our diet.

The best sources of dietary coenzyme Q10 are organ meats, like liver, heart, and kidney, which have high activity rates.

Many vegetarian foods have CoQ10, but it is in such small amounts that it's best to supplement with CoQ10 if you're trying to get pregnant.

Supplementing with CoQ10

Because optimal levels of CoQ10 are difficult to get from food alone, it's easiest to take a supplement.

Ubiquinol is the better absorbed form of CoQ10 whereas Ubiquinone is more commonly found in supplements because of its lower cost.

However, Ubiquinone must be converted to Ubiquinol, so taking Ubiquinol will skip this conversion process.

There is a limit to the amount of CoQ10 that your body will absorb from food or supplements.

Fertility studies that showed a benefit used either 200mg/three times per day or 300mg/twice a day.

Since CoQ10 is fat-soluble, taking it with fatty food also helps with the absorption.

A significantly higher number of primordial follicles was shown after 12 weeks of treatment with CoQ10, so if you choose to supplement with CoQ10, allow at least a three-month trial, if not longer.

Supplementing with DHEA to improve fertility

Dehydroepiandrosterone (DHEA) is a steroid hormone produced mainly in the adrenals and in smaller amounts in the ovaries, testes, skin, and brain.

The adrenals are small, triangular-shaped glands that sit on top of your kidneys, like Pinocchio's hat. In addition to DHEA, the adrenals produce other important hormones, including adrenaline to help your body deal with stress.

In the inactive form, DHEA-S, the DHEA molecule, is bound to a sulfate. This is actually your body's most abundant circulating steroid hormone, and your egg quality depends on having the right amount.

Unfortunately, DHEA levels drop as you age. The concentration of this hormone peaks in your 20s and then begins to naturally decline as you get older.

Why is DHEA important?

DHEA is sometimes called the "mother" hormone because it's a precursor to the major sex steroids (estrogen, progesterone, and testosterone), which are critical for optimal fertility.

DHEA is formed initially from cholesterol, which is converted to pregnenolone, before being transformed to DHEA.

Your body can then use the DHEA to create both androgens, such as testosterone, and estrogens. In women before menopause, 50% to 75% of estrogens and the majority of testosterone are produced from DHEA.

Within the ovaries, the androgen hormones play an important role in the immature egg cell being released.

The right amount of DHEA, which creates the right amount of androgen, is important in fertility.

How does DHEA work?

Women with PCOS often have elevated levels of DHEA-S, and women undergoing IVF often have decreased DHEA levels.

Over the past two decades, many IVF clinics have studied and used DHEA in their practices. Understanding how DHEA works and for whom it is a good fit will help you decide if it is a good option for you.

One study reports that DHEA helps with premature ovarian aging in two ways:

- Increasing free IGF-1 (a growth factor hormone) concentrations

- Increasing anti-Müllerian hormone levels.[20]

There have been many clinical trials on DHEA supplementation for women undergoing IVF.

Most of the studies use 75mg/day of DHEA, often broken up into three doses of 25mg each. Trial participants took the DHEA for three to four months before the eggs were harvested.

The majority of the studies show an increase in number of pregnancies and in live birth rates, especially for women with diminished ovarian reserve.[21]

There have also been trials that did not find a statistically significant increase in the pregnancy rate when using IVF.[22] It is important to note, though, that these studies did not find a negative effect from DHEA.

So why is DHEA supplementation effective for some women undergoing IVF and not for all women? It depends on several factors, including age, genetics, and lifestyle. You can't turn back the clock, but you can investigate your genetic and lifestyle factors.

Testing DHEA levels

As part of your fertility workup, get the DHEA-S blood test to measure the amount of DHEA-S in your bloodstream. It's also a valuable test to check how well your adrenal glands are working.

In premenopausal women, 50% of the DHEA in your body is secreted by the adrenals, up to 25% by the ovaries, and the rest by the skin and brain.

Typical normal DHEA-S ranges for females are:

- Ages 30 to 39: 45 to 270 µg/dL or 1.22 to 7.29 µmol/L
- Ages 40 to 49: 32 to 240 µg/dL or 0.86 to 6.48 µmol/L
- Ages 50 to 59: 26 to 200 µg/dL or 0.70 to 5.40 µmol/L

Supplementing with DHEA

Recommended dosage: 25mg, three times a day (total of 75 mgs daily)

DHEA should be taken at least one month before starting medications to stimulate ovaries, ideally for three to four months.

Lifestyle factors that influence DHEA

In addition to the genetic variants that make you unique, your overall lifestyle can also impact your DHEA levels.

By now, you've already experienced how hard chronic stress is on the body. When it comes to your hormones, the adrenal glands are vital. High stress levels can elevate cortisol, which, in turn, can inhibit the production of the steroid hormones.

In fact, one study found that some women who were diagnosed with having POI actually had adrenal insufficiency, which was contributing to the fertility problems. In some of these cases, DHEA supplementation then helped the patients to conceive.[23]

Even something as common as stress at work can affect your DHEA levels. A study found that women who reported higher levels of stress at work had 23% lower DHEA-S measurements.[24]

This is because as you age, DHEA decreases while cortisol levels remain constant or even increase as a response to more lifestyle stress resulting in an increased cortisol/DHEA-S ratio. The unbalanced relationship between the too high cortisol and not enough DHEA-S is serious enough that it can decrease fertility and prematurely age your eggs.

Exercises, such as Tai Chi and yoga, are associated with higher DHEA levels. In fact, a study found that 12 weeks of yoga increased both DHEA and growth hormone levels.

.

CHAPTER 12

Testing Your Nutritional Status

The only way to know for sure what is going on in your body is to do a blood test. Some of these tests may be something that your doctor can order, and your insurance could pay part of the cost.

If your doctor doesn't want to order the tests or insurance won't pay for it, another great option is to order lab tests online on your own.

Let's dig into some of the research-backed blood markers that can make a difference when trying to conceive.

Vitamin D

Having adequate vitamin D levels is important for overall health as well as reproductive health. While your body can make vitamin D from sun exposure on your skin, so many of us today don't get an adequate amount of sunlight during the day.

The U.S. National Institute of Health recommends that people have vitamin D levels of 20 to 50 ng/mL. But for women trying to conceive, 20 ng/mL may be too low. Studies of women undergoing IVF found that those having vitamin D levels greater than 30 ng/mL were more likely to conceive.[1] Other studies point to 40ng/mL as being important for a healthy pregnancy.[2]

Putting those together, target a minimum level of 30ng/mL when trying to conceive. Once pregnant, aim for least 40ng/mL. Levels should not exceed 60ng/mL.

Raising your vitamin D levels

Getting outside in the sunshine each day is a great way to naturally raise your vitamin D levels. But for people who can't spend enough time outside with their skin exposed to the sun, vitamin D3 is available as a supplement. Look for one based in coconut oil or another healthy oil rather than soy oil.

Excess vitamin D from supplements can cause high serum calcium concentrations. You want to take enough vitamin D to increase your levels to the sweet spot. Retest again after a few months of supplementing to see what your levels are. The Endocrine Society recommends higher doses of up to 50,000 IU/week for eight weeks for women who have vitamin D deficiency.

Vitamin A

Having enough vitamin A is essential when trying to conceive. Studies point to decreased fertility with vitamin A deficiency, and higher levels of retinol (vitamin A) increase the quality of embryos in IVF. One study on in-vitro fertilization found that vitamin A intake of over 700 mcg/day was associated with higher quality embryos.[3]

You may think that you are getting plenty of vitamin A by eating carrots, sweet potatoes, and other sources of beta-carotene. But some people have genetic variants that decrease their ability to convert those plant forms of vitamin A into the retnol form the body needs, so you may be eating plenty of beta-carotene but still not have enough true vitamin A in your cells.

The best way to know your vitamin A status is to get a blood test.

Retinol levels below 20 mcg/dL are considered *sub-clinical vitamin A deficiency.* This is the point where many people may experience problems, such as poor night vision, greater susceptibility to getting sick, and skin problems.

Raising your vitamin A levels

Foods that have a high level of the retinol form of vitamin A include liver, butter from grass-fed cows, and cod liver oil. Supplemental vitamin A is also available. Keep in mind that vitamin A is something that you don't want to go overboard on when trying to conceive. Extremely high doses of retinol can be detrimental to a baby and cause birth defects.

Folate and homocysteine levels

Folate is essential for a healthy baby, and most women are aware of the need for folate in their prenatal vitamins.

A common genetic variant of the MTHFR gene can cause you to need more folate, especially when trying to conceive. Women who carry two copies of the MTHFR C677T variant are more likely to have problems with conception.[4]

Folate is needed within the methylation cycle, which is a biochemical way that your body creates methyl groups for use in various reactions. Methylation is important in detoxification of certain toxins, creation of neurotransmitters, making antioxidants, and more.

If you have been taking prenatal vitamins, you likely will show up as having more than adequate folate on a serum blood test, but this doesn't always tell you how well your body is using the circulating folate and folic acid.

One way to know whether you're having problems with the methylation cycle, though, is by testing homocysteine. Higher than normal homocysteine levels indicate problems with methylation.

Homocysteine is often measured as a marker of heart disease risk, but it is also important when trying to conceive. High homocysteine levels are tied to lower pregnancy rates in IVF.[5]

An inexpensive blood test can show you if your homocysteine level is high. Normal homocysteine levels are less than 10 umol/L for women.[6]

Raising your folate and lowering homocysteine

A diet rich in folate includes broccoli, asparagus, eggs, leafy greens, and liver. If you choose to supplement with folate, look for a methylfolate supplement, which is the active form that your body uses. If your homocysteine levels are high, be sure that you get plenty of riboflavin, B6, folate, and B12 either through diet or supplements.

Optimal thyroid health

Ellen's Story

With symptoms such as low energy, difficulty losing weight, and low sex drive, I suspected that Ellen had a thyroid that wasn't functionally optimally. I explained to Ellen that her TSH level, although normal, wasn't enough to assess her thyroid function.

She was able to convince her doctor to get the full thyroid panel I recommended. Her TSH and Free T3 levels came back normal but on the very low end of the range.

121

Knowing that a higher level would be more ideal, I recommended dietary changes and supplements to support her thyroid. Gradually her symptoms improved, and another blood test confirmed a rise in both her TSH and Free T3 levels.

She was able to get pregnant six months later with a healthy baby boy.

Optimal thyroid health is so important for both your overall well-being and conception.

Women with hypothyroidism are more likely to have problems with infertility.[7]

A standard blood test from your doctor usually includes thyroid stimulating hormone (TSH) as a way to check for thyroid health. But testing TSH only tells you whether your pituitary is signaling for more thyroid hormone to be produced. It doesn't tell you what your thyroid levels actually are.

For a more comprehensive evaluation of your thyroid, have the following tested instead:

- TSH

- Free T3

- Free T4

- TPO (thyroid peroxidase) antibodies

- Tg (thyroglobulin) antibodies

Triiodothyronine (T3) and thyroxine (T4) are the two major thyroid hormones. They are mostly bound to protein in the blood so are inactive. The rest is free, or unbound, and is the biologically active form. Measuring free T3 and free T4 levels may provide a more accurate picture of thyroid function.

Elevated antibody levels may indicate an autoimmune thyroid issue, such as Hashimoto's thyroiditis where the immune system attacks the thyroid. Autoimmune thyroid disease is relatively common, occurring in up to 20% of the U.S. population.

CHAPTER 13

What About Your Partner?

Sperm are, of course, an essential part of getting pregnant.

Many recent studies show that sperm count and sperm quality are declining in many men.

One European study sums up this decline. The study looked at the sperm quality of 10,000+ different men over two decades. The results showed that in the last 20 years, there was a population-wide decline in sperm concentration of 1.5% per year and an increase in abnormal sperm each year.[1]

Another study in the U.S. using 9,000 sperm bank samples also found a significant decline over a ten-year period in both sperm concentration and motility.[2]

What can you do about sperm quality?

Almost all of the lifestyle and dietary changes that have been discussed here also positively affect sperm quality. The saying "what's good for the goose is good for the gander" applies here!

Putting pressure on your male partner to make a lot of changes may backfire on you, though. Reducing stress, including relationship stress, is important. Instead, making the changes outlined here for yourself first will have a trickle-down effect on male sperm quality.

Take phthalate exposure for example. A quick search of studies on phthalate exposure and sperm turns up several thousand research studies on the topic. These studies show:

- Phthalate metabolites in the urine correspond to lower sperm count and a higher number of sperm that are abnormal.[3]

- A recent study of men who were taking a medication that contained phthalates in the coating found that they had a 30 to 71% increase in the odds of having poor semen quality.[4]

The same principle holds true for exposure to BPA and other toxicants. Sleeping well and increasing melatonin is important for sperm quality too.[5]

Lifestyle changes that will also affect sperm quality include:

- Getting rid of the phthalates, BPA, and parabens in your personal care products, laundry detergents, and food storage containers.

- Moderate exercise, such as taking a walk together every evening, will positively impact fertility.

- Losing a little weight together, as a couple, if you both are overweight.

- Prioritize a routine bedtime and decrease the amount of blue light you and everyone in your household is exposed to at night.

Antioxidant rich foods and high-quality dietary choices are important for sperm quality as well. A number of studies show that increasing antioxidants, getting adequate omega-3 fats from fish and seafood, and decreasing consumption of trans fats—all improve sperm quality.[6]

Dietary changes will have a positive effect on sperm quality:

- Simple changes, such as cooking at home rather than eating out all the time.

- Making your meals with high quality protein sources and lots of antioxidant rich, fresh vegetables.

- Choosing organic whenever possible for the foods you buy at the grocery store.

Chasing down your man – a reality check

The reality is that for most couples, it's the woman who take most of the supplements as a proactive measure to improve their chances of getting pregnant.

In general, men are not as compliant about supplementing as women are. From what I've observed, some of the reasons are:

- o *The benefits of the supplements aren't clearly understood.*

- o *Taking supplements are thought of as a nuisance and so they don't want to be bothered.*

- o *They're not a priority in his daily to-do list.*

- o *Taking supplements is an admission that there's something wrong with him.*

Because of how hard it is to get men to take supplements, women often have to chase their men down and almost force feed them.

If you're doing this, my advice is to stop and let it go.

On your fertility journey, your primary goal is to take care of yourself. Period. End of story.

You have no control over anyone else, especially your partner. Your role is to be his partner, lover, and wife, not his mother, or a nag.

By all means, give him the information he needs so he can make an informed decision. Request gently that you would appreciate having him be part of the journey with you by taking supplements to improve sperm quality. Despite what he might think, there's always room for improvement since there's no such thing as perfect sperm.

But recognize that he's an adult and whatever decision he makes, given the information he has, is completely up to him. Let him do his own thing. If he asks for help with keeping the supplements straight, then help him. But that is the extent of your role regarding his supplements.

As much as you know it will help him, he can only implement changes when he's ready, not when you say it's time.

Instead, focus on yourself so that you can be the best version of yourself—the creative, fertile woman you are born to be. That's a journey worth your time and attention, not the angst of what others do or don't do.

In time, as you make your own changes and share your improvements, he may be more motivated to incorporate your suggestions into his lifestyle.

CHAPTER 14

Conclusion and Action Plan

Bottom line: Your fertility can be improved with mindful practices, regardless of your age or diagnosis. There is no one-size-fits-all approach to getting pregnant into your 40s. What works for one woman may not work for another. However, adhering to general guidelines as described above will significantly improve your overall health and, therefore, your fertility.

Create a daily routine using some of the most easily implemented suggested actions. As you get comfortable incorporating the changes, add more according to what suits you.

The point is not to stuff your day with a task list of things to improve your fertility. Instead, identify things you can do that make you feel better. Expect it to be a process of trial and error. You may not necessarily feel better physically with the changes. Rather, they may just provide a sense of ease in knowing that you're making more informed choices. And let that be enough.

.

CHAPTER 15

Recipes

Healthy babies need healthy nutrients. Use these simple and quick recipes for an easy transition to a more nutrient-dense eating plan. All recipes require less than 30 minutes of hands-on cooking and/or prep.

Although not noted specifically in the recipes for ease of reading, buy organic whenever possible.

Bone Broth

- Prep time: 2 minutes
- Cook time: overnight and longer

Ingredients

- Bones (choose one or a mixture):
  - Grass-fed beef bones
  - Pastured chicken bones
  - Available at a natural health foods store, farmers market, or online

- Dried kelp
  - A natural source of iodine for healthy thyroid function
  - Available at Asian markets, natural health foods store, or online

- Generous splash of apple cider vinegar

- Lots of filtered water

How to Make Bone Broth

1. Cover the bottom of the slow cooker insert with a layer of bones, a few pieces of kelp, and a generous splash of apple cider vinegar.

2. Optional: add herbs and veggies for additional flavor. You're not getting many nutrients from the veggies because they're cooked for so long.

3. Add filtered water to the top of slow cooker.

4. Cook at the lowest setting overnight.

5. Optional: In the morning, place stoneware in refrigerator until fat solidifies to be skimmed off. Keep fat for cooking. Put stoneware back into slow cooker. Select lowest setting.

6. Serve as needed. Salt to taste.

7. Add more water to slow cooker as you take out what you need.

8. Keep slow cooker on lowest setting. The longer it cooks, the more it releases the marrow, collagen, minerals, and other nutrients. Important! Make sure the broth continues to simmer to prevent bacterial growth.

9. Use bones until bone broth loses flavor or bones crumble easily. One batch of bones can last several days, depending on how much you drink.

Tip:

- Save vegetables scraps in the freezer to add to your bone broth. Stuff like, ends of carrots, onion peels, chunks of tomato, celery leaves and ends.

Bone Broth Green Smoothie

- Prep time: 5 minutes
- Cook time: none
- Total time: 5 minutes
- Servings: 1

Ingredients

- 2 cups bone broth (homemade or pre-made)
- 2 handfuls of dark leafy greens like spinach or kale
- Cilantro, a few sprigs (optional)
- Sea salt

Directions

1. Blend first three ingredients in blender.

2. Salt to taste.

3. Pour into heat-proof mug. Serve with hard-boiled eggs for a quick meal.

Tip:

Prepare a bunch of hard-boiled eggs on the weekend so that you can grab from the refrigerator whenever hunger strikes or to pack a meal quickly.

Butternut Squash Soup

- Prep time: 10 minutes
- Cook time: 45 minutes
- Total time: 55 minutes
- Servings: 4

Ingredients:

- 1 large butternut squash
- 4 raw eggs
- ½ c bone broth or water
- 1 avocado
- 3 tbsp butter or coconut oil
- Salt (to taste)

Instructions:

1. Prepare butternut squash.

- Preheat oven to 375° F.

- Cut butternut squash in half lengthwise.

- Place cut side down on parchment paper on cookie sheet.

- Bake for about 45 minutes or until tender.

- Let cool.

- Using a spoon, remove seeds and string to discard.

- Scoop out flesh into blender or food processor.

2. Add remaining ingredients into blender and blend well.

3. Add salt to taste.

Note:

To make this recipe vegan or vegetarian, replace butter with coconut oil and omit eggs.

Broccoli "Cheese" Soup

- Prep time: 10 minutes
- Cook time: 20 minutes
- Total time: 30 minutes
- Servings: 4

Ingredients:

- 2 tablespoons coconut oil
- ½ onion , diced
- 1-2 cloves garlic , minced
- 3 cups bone broth + more to thin out soup
- 4 cups broccoli florets
- 1 ½ cups shredded carrot , about 2 medium
- 1 cup raw cashews , soaked for 4 hours
- ½ teaspoon mustard powder or 1 tsp prepared mustard
- ½ teaspoon smoked paprika
- ½ cup nutritional yeast (provides the cheesy flavor)
- 1 tablespoon fresh lemon juice , about half a lemon
- Cayenne pepper, dash
- Sea salt
- Freshly cracked pepper
- Cooked pasture-raised bacon pieces (optional)
- Avocado, diced (optional)

Instructions

1. In a medium saucepan over medium heat, heat coconut oil. Add onion and sauté until translucent, stirring often. Add garlic and cook, stirring constantly, about 30 seconds, or until fragrant.

2. Add 2 cups bone broth, broccoli, and carrots. Cover with a lid. Simmer until broccoli is tender, about 6-8 minutes.

3. In a blender, combine cashews, water, mustard powder, smoked paprika, nutritional yeast, lemon juice, 1 cup bone broth, and cayenne pepper. Blend at high speed until very smooth.

4. Add broccoli mixture to blender and pulse a few times to incorporate, keeping small pieces of vegetables intact for texture.

5. Add sea salt and freshly cracked pepper to taste.

6. Thin out with bone broth to desired consistency. Spoon into serving bowls. Top with bacon and avocado.

Creamy Broccoli "Polenta"

- Prep time: 5 minutes
- Cook time: 15 minutes
- Total time: 20 minutes
- Servings: 2

Ingredients:

- 1 bag cauliflower or broccoli florets
- 3 tbsp nutritional yeast
- 2 garlic cloves, minced
- 1 tbsp butter/ghee/or coconut oil
- 1 tsp sea salt
- ¼ tsp black pepper
- 1 cup bone broth or water

Directions

1. Bring a large pot with bone broth to a boil.

2. Add the florets and reduce the heat to medium-low.

3. Boil for 10 minutes.

4. Drain the florets and reserve the liquid.

5. Add cooked florets, ¼ cup reserved bone broth, and ingredients 2-6 to a blender or food processor. Blend until creamy.

6. Serve immediately topped with desired sauce such as meat sauce.

French Toast Fake-Out

Miss the decadence of french toast? Try this recipe using eggplant, instead of bread. Microwave the eggplant first to reduce its distinctive taste. Adding a topping will further neutralize the eggplant and add decadence.

- Prep time: 5 minutes
- Cook time: 10 minutes
- Total time: 15 minutes
- Servings: 3

Ingredients:

- 1 eggplant, peeled and sliced about ½" thick
- 2 eggs, beaten
- Pinch of salt
- Grass-fed butter/ghee or organic coconut oil

Directions:

1. Microwave each eggplant slice 30-45 seconds. You want the eggplant to be cooked through but not so mushy that it breaks apart when handled. Experiment with a few slices to get the right cooking time.

2. Add a pinch of salt to beaten eggs.

3. Soak eggplant in egg. Turn eggplant over to soak other side in egg.

4. Melt butter in non-stick pan over medium heat.

5. Place eggplant in pan and cook until golden brown, about 1 minute.

6. Turn eggplant over to cook other side until golden brown, about 1 minute.

7. Remove from heat and add toppings.

Topping suggestions:

- Bananas fried in butter
- Nut butter
- Maple syrup
- Raw, local honey
- Shredded, unsweetened coconut
- Fresh berries
- Chopped nuts

Avocado & Egg Sandwich

- Prep time: 1 minute
- Cook time: 5 minutes
- Total time: 6 minutes
- Servings: 1

Ingredients:

- 1 tbsp grass-fed butter
- ¼ tsp baking powder
- 2 tbsp organic coconut flour
- Pinch of sea salt
- 3 tbsp filtered water or bone broth
- Pinch of garlic powder and onion powder (optional)
- 1 pasture-raised egg
- ½ organic avocado, sliced
- For seasoning: salt, pepper, olive oil

Instructions:

1. Melt butter in microwaveable glass or ceramic dish (not plastic!) for about 30 seconds.

2. Stir in baking powder, flour, salt, water, garlic powder, and onion powder until well mixed.

3. Microwave for 3 minutes.

4. Remove bread from dish. Once cooled, slice in half horizontally.

5. Crack an egg into dish. Sprinkle with salt. Beat egg. Microwave for 45 seconds.

6. Top 1 bread half with avocado. Season with salt & pepper. Drizzle with olive oil.

7. Top with egg.

Tuna Salad

- Prep time: 10 minutes
- Cook time: none
- Total time: 10 minutes
- Servings: 2

Ingredients:

- 1 can tuna in water
- 1 tablespoon cilantro, chopped
- 1 tablespoon onion, chopped
- 1 avocado, mashed
- lemon
- Salt
- Pepper
- Lettuce cups or endive

Instructions:

1. In a bowl, mix the first 4 ingredients with a squeeze of lemon

2. Add salt & pepper to taste.

3. Spoon tuna salad into lettuce cups.

Superfood Chocolate Smoothie

- Prep time: 5 minutes
- Cook time: none
- Total time: 5 minutes
- Serving: 1

Ingredients:

- 1 ½ tbsp. organic, raw cacao powder (NOT the same as cocoa powder which is more processed)
- 1 tbsp organic maca powder
- 1 raw organic, pastured egg or 1 scoop grass-fed collagen powder
- Handful of spinach
- ¼ quarter organic avocado
- pinch cinnamon powder
- pinch ginger powder or grated fresh organic ginger
- Liquid stevia to taste

Directions:

1. Blend all ingredients with a few cubes of ice. Add cold water (or bone broth) to desired consistency. Try freezing bone broth into ice cubes to add even more nutrients than just plain water! Anywhere you can add bone broth, do so.

2. Serve immediately.

Chia Seed Pudding

- Prep time: 5 minutes
- Inactive time: 4 hours
- Total time: 4 hours 5 minutes
- Serving: 2

Ingredients

- ⅔ cup full fat coconut milk
- ⅓ cup water
- 3 tbsp chia seed
- ½ tsp Almond or vanilla extract
- Liquid stevia, to taste (don't need this if topping with fruit)

Directions

1. Add coconut milk, water, and extract into glass container. Whisk in chia seeds. Add liquid stevia to taste.

2. Pour mixture into a glass container and place in the refrigerator for at least 4 hours or overnight to gel.

3. Whisk a few times within the first hour to help it gel evenly.

4. Top with fruit or nuts.

Variation:

Add 1 tbsp cacao powder for chocolate chia seed pudding.

Liver Pate

- Prep time: 5 minutes
- Cook time: 25 minutes

Ingredients:

- 2 tbsp grass-fed butter or organic coconut oil
- 1 lb chicken livers, rinsed in cold water & drained
- 1 medium onion, sliced
- ½ cooking apple (Granny Smith, Jonagold, Honeycrisp) peeled, cored and chopped
- ½ tsp sea salt
- ½ tsp pepper
- Ground nutmeg (optional)
- ½ cup bone broth (or full fat coconut milk or water)

Instructions:

1. Melt coconut oil in pan over medium high heat.

2. Add sliced onions and cook, stirring occasionally, until they become soft and golden, about 10 minutes. Add a few tablespoons of bone broth if onions get too brown or start sticking to the pan.

3. When the onions are soft and golden, add apple to the pan. Continue cooking for 4-5 minutes, until the apple gets soft. Again, add a little bit of bone broth if mixture gets too dry.

4. Add the chicken liver to the mixture in the pan. Continue cooking for another 5 minutes or so, until the liver is brown on the outside but still slightly pink on the inside.

5. Transfer the mixture to a blender or food processor. Add salt, pepper, and nutmeg. Blend until smooth, adding bone broth as needed so it can mix easily. Be careful about adding too much liquid since you want it on the thicker side so that it can be spread with a knife. Season with more salt, pepper, and nutmeg to taste.

6. Pour the mixture into a container and refrigerate until ready to eat.

7. This pâté will keep for about 3-4 days in the refrigerator. Freeze any extra. Just transfer it from the freezer to the fridge the night before.

8. Serve pate with baby carrots, radishes, celery, apples, pears, jicama slices. Have extra time? Serve on cucumber slices topped with chopped hard-boiled egg and onion.

Because of liver's strong flavor, it can be an acquired taste for many people. If the liver taste bothers you, here are some things you can do to make it less "livery"...

- soak liver in milk overnight and rinse thoroughly before cooking

- add 1 whole apple instead of ½ apple

- Add hot sauce which should disguise most, if not all, of the taste completely.

.

Summaries

Chapter 2: Fertility Specialists and Testing: Making Sense of the Details

6 science-backed steps that you can take today to raise low AMH levels:

- Eat whole, unprocessed, nutrient-dense foods, such as grass-fed meat, wild fish, pasture-raised eggs, organic vegetables, and healthy fats.

- Avoid fried foods and limit omega-6 oils, such as corn, soybean, and sunflower oils.

- Add in curcumin, either as a supplement or in your foods each day.

- Avoid BPA exposure as much as possible. Don't use plastic containers for warming foods. Check the labels to make sure your canned foods are BPA free. Avoid handling thermal printed receipts as much as possible.

- Stay away from pesticides, such as pyrethroids, which are found in many household insecticides. Choose organic fruits and produce as much as possible.

- Avoid sunscreen or cosmetics with titanium dioxide. Check product labels.

If you are dealing with low AMH levels, stack all of these action steps together. This is the time to go all in to clean up your diet, avoid pesticides and toxins, and add the right nutrients!

Chapter 3: A Diagnosis of Primary Ovarian Insufficiency

5 Steps You Can Take Today to Treat POI:

- Workout: Try a moderate weight lifting workout at the gym. If you aren't a gym member, body weight exercises, such as pushups and squats are easy (and free!) to do at home.

- Schedule some lab tests: The only way to know how well your thyroid is functioning is to get it tested, so call your doctor to schedule an appointment or order your own lab work online.

- Avoid smokers: Make an effort to remove yourself from situations where people will be smoking around you. This may mean taking a walk during lunch instead of hanging out with coworkers who are smoking.

- Eat a healthy diet that includes plenty of folate: Fix a salad for dinner tonight that includes organic dark leafy green veggies topped with grilled steak.

- Stimulate melatonin production: Turn off your electronic devices and turn down the overhead lights for a couple of hours before bed. Reading a book using a table lamp or relaxing in a bathtub surrounded by candles is a great way to wind down before bed while increasing melatonin naturally.

Chapter 4: Enhancing Egg Quality

3 Steps you can take today to boost Nrf2 for antioxidant defense:

- Making time to exercise regularly is important for fertility in many ways. Get into a routine of getting moderate exercise every day. This can be as simple as changing where you park so that you get in a 15-minute brisk walk to and from work. Or you could get some weights and resistance bands to use for a half hour each evening while watching Netflix.

- If your diet isn't abundant in polyphenol-rich foods, you may want to consider supplementing. Try adding curcumin, sulforaphane, or naringenin. While you don't want to go overboard with high doses of antioxidant supplements, most people will benefit from adding antioxidants.

- Even if you choose to supplement, adding foods, such as broccoli and olive oil, are easy ways to boost your Nrf2 and balance your diet. Focus on getting fresh vegetables in your diet each day, and choose organic whenever possible.

5 natural ways to lengthen your telomeres to improve egg quality and reduce DNA damage:

- Cut out sugar sweetened beverages. Swap out your daily soda for an herbal tea.

- Get active. You don't have to go out and jog five miles every day. Moderate activity is enough to lengthen telomeres.

147

- Increase your intake of omega-3 fats by eating mercury-safe fish. Decrease your consumption of omega-6 fats by cutting out fried foods.

- Make sure you are getting enough fiber in your diet. Replace refined carbohydrates (bread, pasta, and packaged foods) with whole foods instead.

- Sleep well. Go to bed at a reasonable hour and focus on getting quality sleep.

5 action steps you can take today to reduce your BPA levels:

- Reduce or completely eliminate canned foods. Switch to fresh or frozen fruits and vegetables.

- Switch from plastic water bottles to glass or stainless steel bottles.

- Cook at home more often. Plan ahead and have some simple meal options, such as vegetables and meat to put on the grill.

- Get 8 to 9 hours of quality sleep and let your melatonin levels rise naturally at night. Blocking out the blue light from electronics and bright overhead lights at night will increase your melatonin levels, protecting your eggs from BPA.

- Stop storing and microwaving your leftovers in plastic, including Styrofoam and lined cardboard boxes. It is time to start collecting glass containers of various sizes to store your hot food.

Chapter 5: Getting Rid of the Toxicants that Decrease the Quality of Your Eggs

5 action steps you can take today to reduce phthalate exposure:

- Check your laundry detergent, fabric softener, and dryer sheets. These often contain artificial fragrances that increase your phthalate exposure. Switch to a natural laundry option that is labeled *free and clear* or contains essential oils for fragrance.

- Add more folate to your diet. Grass-fed beef liver is a great source of folate and other essential vitamins. A 100g serving of liver packs a whopping 212 mcg of folate. Not a liver fan? Eat more dark, leafy green vegetables. Take a methylfolate supplement to ensure adequate levels–800 mcg a day is recommended.

- Go through your cosmetics, hair care products, and lotions. Read the ingredients to see if they contain phthalates. Find replacements for the items that contain ingredients that are likely to be impacting your fertility.

- Get rid of the artificial air fresheners around your house and workspace.

- Break out the dust rag and clean up any household dust that may contain phthalates and BPA.

2 action steps you can take today to reduce paraben exposure:

- Check labels on your personal care products, especially lotions, cosmetics, and sunscreens. Swap out the ones that contain parabens for more natural options. This is a great time to clean out and eliminate all of the personal care products you no longer need. In addition, consider minimizing the number of products you use on your skin and hair.

- Consider switching to a natural deodorant. Not only will you avoid the parabens, but many deodorants also contain phthalates as part of the *fragrance.*

Chapter 6: Improving Mitochondrial Function in Your Eggs

5 Steps you can take today to boost mitochondrial function:

- Make sure you are getting enough CoQ10 in your diet. Foods rich in CoQ10 include organ meats, such as heart and liver, and meats, such as beef and pork. If you aren't getting enough CoQ10 in your diet, consider supplementing.

- Grab your headphones, put on a podcast or some music, and get outside for some exercise today. Moderate, regular exercise will help to increase mitochondrial function.

- Have fatty fish like wild salmon, herring, mackerel, or sardines several times a week. Fish are a great source of both protein and omega-3 fatty acids.

- Go through your medicine cabinet to see if any of the OTC medications you take regularly could be affecting your mitochondria.

- Cut back on sugar and processed carbohydrates to stabilize your insulin levels. Replace sodas and sugar-sweetened drinks with herbal teas and purified water.

Chapter 7: Sleep and Melatonin: A Key to Conception

3 Steps you can take today to boost melatonin:

- Block out blue light at night. Either turn off electronics (TV, laptops, cell phones, tablets) and dim the overhead lighting two hours before bedtime *or* wear blue-blocking glasses that block 100% of the blue light for two hours before bedtime.

- Get some sunlight every morning. Head outside for a walk shortly after the sun comes up. Or drink your coffee on the porch each morning.

- Consider supplementing with low-dose, timed-release melatonin.

Chapter 9: Leptin: A Hormone that Links Your Weight to Fertility

5 steps you can take today to increase your sensitivity to leptin:

- Reduce your triglyceride levels if they are high. Lowering your carbohydrates and specifically avoiding high fructose corn syrup may help to lower triglycerides.

- If you are overweight, try losing weight through a nutrient dense diet that includes organic meats and vegetables.

- Exercise in moderation.

- Sleep well and avoid blue light for two hours before bed.

3 Steps you can take today to get more active:

- Get up and move around for a few minutes every hour. If you have an activity monitor, like a Fitbit or Oura ring, set it so that it reminds you hourly to move if you haven't. Otherwise, set a reminder on your cell phone. Get up and walk around the office, do some air squats, take a dance break—just move!

- Get others in your office involved as well. It makes it so much easier to be accountable and not look foolish if everyone is moving each hour, too.

- Get in the habit of parking farther away from stores and the office. You will get more exercise, and you will leave those front parking spots available for an elderly person who needs it.

Chapter 10:

4 Important Lifestyle changes you can start today:

- Get rid of toxicants. Read the ingredients on your personal care products to see if they contain phthalates or parabens. Toss the products that you don't really need, like lotions you received as a holiday gift. Then find healthier alternatives for what you use on a daily basis.

- Start an exercise routine. Often it is easier to stick to a moderate exercise routine if you involve a friend for accountability, so make today the day that you recruit a friend for a daily hour-long walk. First thing in the morning is great for the early day sunlight exposure, but walking with a co-worker may be more convenient. An after-dinner walk with your partner is an excellent way to reconnect after a long day.

- Take a realistic look at what is causing you stress. Is it your job? Relationship with family or friends? Does your daily commute start your day with a lot of stress? Decide on one step you can take today to decrease your stress. If it is a relationship, perhaps backing off on communicating with that person (mute them on Facebook, stop following on Instagram) is needed at this time in your life.

- Nature is a powerful way to reduce stress, and one that we often don't think about in our busy lives. Schedule some down time this week and go for a short hike in a nearby forest. Live in the heart of a big city? Spend some time in a park, botanical garden, or greenway.

Additional Resources

- To learn more about Julie's other products and programs, visit *FertilityEggspurt.com.*

- American Board of Oriental Reproductive Medicine (ABORM) is an international organization pioneering best practices in acupuncture and oriental reproductive medicine.

- American Society for Reproductive Medicine (ASRM) is a multidisciplinary organization dedicated to the advancement of the art, science, and practice of reproductive medicine.

- RESOLVE: The National Infertility Association is dedicated to ensuring that all people challenged in their family building journey reach resolution.

- Weston A. Price Foundation is dedicated to restoring nutrient-dense foods to the human diet through education, research and activism.

-

References

Chapter 1: Why is Getting Pregnant More Difficult Now?

1. National Summary Report. https://www.sartcorsonline.com/rptCSR_PublicMultYear.aspx?reportingYear=2017.

Chapter 2: Fertility Specialists and Testing: Making Sense of the Details

1. Cui, Yuqian, et al. "Age-Specific Serum Antimüllerian Hormone Levels in Women with and without Polycystic Ovary Syndrome." *Fertility and Sterility*, vol. 102, no. 1, July 2014, pp. 230-236.

2. Hagen, Casper P., et al. "Low Concentration of Circulating Antimüllerian Hormone Is Not Predictive of Reduced Fecundability in Young Healthy Women: A Prospective Cohort Study." *Fertility and Sterility*, vol. 98, no. 6, Dec. 2012, pp. 1602-1608.

3. Koo, Hwa Seon, et al. "The Likelihood of Achieving Pregnancy through Timed Coitus in Young Infertile Women with Decreased Ovarian Reserve." *Clinical and*

Experimental Reproductive Medicine, vol. 45, no. 1, Mar. 2018, pp. 31–37.

4. Hvidman, Helene W., et al. "Anti-Müllerian Hormone Levels and Fecundability in Women with a Natural Conception." *European Journal of Obstetrics, Gynecology, and Reproductive Biology* , vol. 217, Oct. 2017, pp. 44–52.

5. Yan, Zhengjie, et al. "Curcumin Exerts a Protective Effect against Premature Ovarian Failure in Mice." *Journal of Molecular Endocrinology*, vol. 60, no. 3, 2018, pp. 261–71.

6. Xie, Li, et al. "Huyang Yangkun Formula Protects against 4-Vinylcyclohexene Diepoxide-Induced Premature Ovarian Insufficiency in Rats via the Hippo–JAK2/STAT3 Signaling Pathway." *Biomedicine & Pharmacotherapy*, vol. 116, Aug. 2019, p. 109008.

7. Tan, Li, et al. "Chinese Herbal Medicine for Infertility with Anovulation: A Systematic Review." *Journal of Alternative and Complementary Medicine (New York, N.Y.)*, vol. 18, no. 12, Dec. 2012, pp. 1087–100.

8. Teng, Benqi, et al. "Successful Pregnancy after Treatment with Chinese Herbal Medicine in a 43-Year-Old Woman with Diminished Ovarian Reserve and Multiple Uterus Fibrosis: A Case Report." *Medicines*, vol. 4, no. 1, Feb. 2017.

9. "Effect of Chinese Herbal Medicine on Female Infertility." *Obstetrics & Gynecology International Journal*, Volume 8, Issue 1, Sept. 2017.

10. Vincentelli, Clara, et al. "One-Year Impact of Bariatric Surgery on Serum anti-Müllerian-Hormone Levels in Severely Obese Women." *Journal of Assisted Reproduction and Genetics*, vol. 35, no. 7, July 2018, pp. 1317–24. *PubMed*, doi:10.1007/s10815-018-1196-3.

11. Anderson, Chelsea, et al. "Dietary Factors and Serum Antimüllerian Hormone Concentrations in Late Premenopausal Women." *Fertility and Sterility*, vol. 110, no. 6, 2018, pp. 1145–53.

12. Cakmak, Erol, et al. "Ovarian Reserve Assessment in Celiac Patients of Reproductive Age." *Medical Science Monitor: International Medical Journal of Experimental and Clinical Research* , vol. 24, Feb. 2018, pp. 1152–57.

13. Şenateş, Ebubekir, et al. "Serum Anti-Müllerian Hormone Levels Are Lower in Reproductive-Age Women with Crohn's Disease Compared to Healthy Control Women." *Journal of Crohn's & Colitis*, vol. 7, no. 2, Mar. 2013, pp. e29-34.

14. Souter, Irene, et al. "The Association of Bisphenol-A Urinary Concentrations with Antral Follicle Counts and Other Measures of Ovarian Reserve in Women Undergoing Infertility Treatments." *Reproductive Toxicology (Elmsford, N.Y.)*, vol. 42, Dec. 2013, pp. 224–31.

15. Zhou, Wei, et al. "Bisphenol A and Ovarian Reserve among Infertile Women with Polycystic Ovarian Syndrome." *International Journal of Environmental Research and Public Health*, vol. 14, no. 1, Jan. 2017.

16. W, Pan, et al. "Selected Persistent Organic Pollutants Associated With the Risk of Primary Ovarian Insufficiency in Women." *Environment International*, Aug. 2019.

17. Whitworth, Kristina W., et al. "Anti-Müllerian Hormone and Lifestyle, Reproductive, and Environmental Factors among Women in Rural South Africa." *Epidemiology (Cambridge, Mass.)*, vol. 26, no. 3, May 2015, pp. 429–35.

18. Hong, Fashui, and Ling Wang. "Nanosized Titanium Dioxide-Induced Premature Ovarian Failure Is Associated with Abnormalities in Serum Parameters in Female Mice." *International Journal of Nanomedicine*, vol. 13, 2018, pp. 2543–49.

19. E, Al-Eisa, et al. "Effects of Supervised Aerobic Training on the Levels of anti-Müllerian Hormone and Adiposity Measures in Women With Normo-Ovulatory and Polycystic Ovary Syndrome." *JPMA. The Journal of the Pakistan Medical Association*, Apr. 2017.

Chapter 3: A Diagnosis of Primary Ovarian Insufficiency

1. "What Are My Family Planning Options If I Have POI?" http://www.nichd.nih.gov/health/topics/poi/conditioni nfo/family_options.

2. Sun, Xinhui, et al. "New Strategy for in Vitro Activation of Primordial Follicles with MTOR and PI3K Stimulators." *Cell Cycle (Georgetown, Tex.)*, vol. 14, no. 5, 2015, pp. 721–31.

3. Dalle Pezze, Piero, et al. "A Systems Study Reveals Concurrent Activation of AMPK and MTOR by Amino Acids." *Nature Communications*, vol. 7, 21 2016, p. 13254.

4. Blomstrand, Eva, et al. "Branched-Chain Amino Acids Activate Key Enzymes in Protein Synthesis after Physical Exercise." *The Journal of Nutrition*, vol. 136, no. 1 Suppl, 2006, pp. 269S-73S.

5. Goyco Ortiz, Luz E., et al. "A Successful Treatment with 5 Methyltetrahydrofolate of a 677 TT MTHFR Woman Suffering Premature Ovarian Insufficiency Post a NHL (Non-Hodgkin's Lymphoma) and RPL (Repeat Pregnancy Losses)." *Journal of Assisted Reproduction and Genetics*, vol. 36, no. 1, Jan. 2019, pp. 65–67.

6. Bakalov, Vladimir K., et al. "Autoimmune Disorders in Women with Turner Syndrome and Women with Karyotypically Normal Primary Ovarian Insufficiency." *Journal of Autoimmunity*, vol. 38, no. 4, June 2012, pp. 315–21.

7. Zhu, Dongshan, et al. "Relationships between Intensity, Duration, Cumulative Dose, and Timing of Smoking with Age at Menopause: A Pooled Analysis of Individual Data from 17 Observational Studies."

8. Chen, Yingru, et al. "Effect of Acupuncture on Premature Ovarian Failure: A Pilot Study."*Evidence-Based Complementary and Alternative Medicine* : ECAM, vol. 2014, 2014.

9. Ma, Min, et al. "Melatonin Protects Premature Ovarian Insufficiency Induced by Tripterygium Glycosides: Role of SIRT1." *American Journal of Translational Research*, vol. 9, no. 4, Apr. 2017, pp. 1580–602.

10. Ostrin, Lisa A., et al. "Attenuation of Short Wavelengths Alters Sleep and the IpRGC Pupil Response." *Ophthalmic & Physiological Optics: The Journal of the British College of Ophthalmic Opticians (Optometrists)*, vol. 37, no. 4, 2017, pp. 440–50.

Chapter 4: Enhancing Your Egg Quality

1. Tomza-Marciniak, Agnieszka, et al. "Effect of Bisphenol A on Reproductive Processes: A Review of in Vitro, in Vivo and Epidemiological Studies." *Journal of Applied Toxicology: JAT*, vol. 38, no. 1, Jan. 2018, pp. 51–80.

2. Jahromi, Bahia Namavar, et al. "Effect of Melatonin on the Outcome of Assisted Reproductive Technique Cycles in Women with Diminished Ovarian Reserve: A Double-Blinded Randomized Clinical Trial." *Iranian Journal of Medical Sciences*, vol. 42, no. 1, Jan. 2017, pp. 73–78.

3. Keefe, David L., and Lin Liu. "Telomeres and Reproductive Aging." *Reproduction, Fertility, and Development*, vol. 21, no. 1, 2009, pp. 10–14.

4. Keefe, David L. "Telomeres, Reproductive Aging, and Genomic Instability During Early Development." *Reproductive Sciences (Thousand Oaks, Calif.)*, vol. 23, no. 12, 2016, pp. 1612–15.

5. Bhaumik, Pranami, et al. "Telomere Length Analysis in Down Syndrome Birth." *Mechanisms of Ageing and Development*, vol. 164, 2017, pp. 20–26.

6. Ray, Anirban, et al. "Maternal Telomere Length and Risk of Down Syndrome: Epidemiological Impact of Smokeless Chewing Tobacco and Oral Contraceptive on Segregation of Chromosome 21." *Public Health Genomics*, vol. 19, no. 1, 2016, pp. 11–18.

7. Astuti, Yuliana, et al. "Cigarette Smoking and Telomere Length: A Systematic Review of 84 Studies and Meta-Analysis." *Environmental Research*, vol. 158, 2017, pp. 480–89.

8. Du, Mengmeng, et al. "Physical Activity, Sedentary Behavior, and Leukocyte Telomere Length in Women." *American Journal of Epidemiology*, vol. 175, no. 5, Mar. 2012, pp. 414–22.

9. Kiecolt-Glaser, Janice K., et al. "Omega-3 Fatty Acids, Oxidative Stress, and Leukocyte Telomere Length: A Randomized Controlled Trial." *Brain, Behavior, and Immunity*, vol. 28, Feb. 2013, pp. 16–24.

10. Wynchank, Dora, et al. "Delayed Sleep-Onset and Biological Age: Late Sleep-Onset Is Associated with Shorter Telomere Length." *Sleep*, vol. 42, no. 10, Oct. 2019.

11. Leung, Cindy W., et al. "Soda and Cell Aging: Associations Between Sugar-Sweetened Beverage Consumption and Leukocyte Telomere Length in Healthy Adults From the National Health and Nutrition Examination Surveys." *American Journal of Public Health*, vol. 104, no. 12, Dec. 2014, pp. 2425–31.

12. Tucker, Larry A. "Dietary Fiber and Telomere Length in 5674 U.S. Adults: An NHANES Study of Biological Aging." *Nutrients*, vol. 10, no. 4, Mar. 2018.

13. Kiecolt-Glaser, Janice K., et al. "Omega-3 Fatty Acids, Oxidative Stress, and Leukocyte Telomere Length: A Randomized Controlled Trial." *Brain, Behavior, and Immunity*, vol. 28, Feb. 2013, pp. 16–24.

14. Tamura, Hiroshi, et al. "Long-Term Melatonin Treatment Delays Ovarian Aging." *Journal of Pineal Research*, vol. 62, no. 2, Mar. 2017.

15. Yu, Yongjie, et al. "Cycloastragenol: An Exciting Novel Candidate for Age-Associated Diseases." *Experimental and Therapeutic Medicine*, vol. 16, no. 3, Sept. 2018, pp. 2175–82.

16. Tarín, J. J. "Potential Effects of Age-Associated Oxidative Stress on Mammalian Oocytes/Embryos." *Molecular Human Reproduction*, vol. 2, no. 10, Oct. 1996, pp. 717–24.

17. Ou, Xiang-Hong, et al. "Maternal Insulin Resistance Causes Oxidative Stress and Mitochondrial Dysfunction in Mouse Oocytes." *Human Reproduction (Oxford, England)*, vol. 27, no. 7, July 2012, pp. 2130–45.

18. Zhao, Jun, et al. "Pre-Pregnancy Maternal Fasting Plasma Glucose Levels in Relation to Time to Pregnancy among the Couples Attempting First Pregnancy." *Human Reproduction (Oxford, England)*, vol. 34, no. 7, July 2019, pp. 1325–33.

19. Terao, Hiromi, et al. "Role of Oxidative Stress in Follicular Fluid on Embryos of Patients Undergoing Assisted Reproductive Technology Treatment." *The Journal of Obstetrics and Gynaecology Research*, vol. 45, no. 9, Sept. 2019, pp. 1884–91.

20. Mihalas, Bettina P., et al. "Molecular Mechanisms Responsible for Increased Vulnerability of the Ageing Oocyte to Oxidative Damage." *Oxidative Medicine and Cellular Longevity*, vol. 2017, 2017.

21. Kumar, Sunil, et al. "Role of Environmental Factors & Oxidative Stress with Respect to in Vitro Fertilization Outcome." *The Indian Journal of Medical Research*, vol. 148, no. Suppl 1, Dec. 2018, pp. S125–33.

22. Li, Zhichao, et al. "Preincubation with Glutathione Ethyl Ester Improves the Developmental Competence of Vitrified Mouse Oocytes." *Journal of Assisted Reproduction and Genetics*, vol. 35, no. 7, July 2018, pp. 1169–78.

23. Mokhtari, Vida, et al. "A Review on Various Uses of N-Acetyl Cysteine." *Cell Journal (Yakhteh)*, vol. 19, no. 1, 2017, pp. 11–17.

24. Harada, Miwa, et al. "Infertility Observed in Reproductive Toxicity Study of N-Acetyl-L-Cysteine in Rats." *Biology of Reproduction*, vol. 69, no. 1, July 2003, pp. 242–47.

25. Sarutipaiboon, Ingkarat, et al. "Association of Genetic Variations in NRF2, NQO1, HMOX1, and MT with Severity of Coronary Artery Disease and Related Risk Factors." *Cardiovascular Toxicology*, July 2019. *PubMed*, doi:10.1007/s12012-019-09544-7.

26. Kala, Manika, et al. "Equilibrium between Anti-oxidants and Reactive Oxygen Species: A Requisite for Oocyte Development and Maturation." Reproductive Medicine and Biology, vol. 16, no. 1, Dec. 2016, pp. 28–35.

27. Agarwal, Ashok, et al. "Oxidative Stress and Its Implications in Female Infertility - a Clinician's Perspective." Reproductive Biomedicine Online, vol. 11, no. 5, Nov. 2005, pp. 641–50.

28. Qiu, X., and B. Yao. "Nrf2 Regulates Female Germ Cell Meiosis Initiation." *Fertility and Sterility*, vol. 108, no. 3, Sept. 2017, p. e153.

29. Akino, Nana, et al. "Activation of Nrf2/Keap1 Pathway by Oral Dimethylfumarate Administration Alleviates Oxidative Stress and Age-Associated Infertility Might Be Delayed in the Mouse Ovary." *Reproductive Biology and Endocrinology*, vol. 17, no. 1, Feb. 2019, p. 23.

30. Hussain, Tarique, et al. Modulatory Mechanism of Polyphenols and Nrf2 Signaling Pathway in LPS Challenged Pregnancy Disorders. Oxidative Medicine and Cellular Longevity, Vol. 2017, Article ID 8254289, 14 pages.

31. Vargas-Mendoza, Nancy, et al. "Antioxidant and Adaptative Response Mediated by Nrf2 during Physical Exercise." *Antioxidants*, vol. 8, no. 6, June 2019. *PubMed Central*, doi:10.3390/antiox8060196.

32. Yan, Zhengjie, et al. "Curcumin Exerts a Protective Effect against Premature Ovarian Failure in Mice." Journal of Molecular Endocrinology, vol. 60, no. 3, Feb. 2018, pp. 261–71.

33. Kapoor, Radhika, et al. "Naringenin Ameliorates Progression of Endometriosis by Modulating

Nrf2/Keap1/HO1 Axis and Inducing Apoptosis in Rats." *The Journal of Nutritional Biochemistry*, vol. 70, Aug. 2019, pp. 215–26. *PubMed*, doi:10.1016/j.jnutbio.2019.05.003.

34. Dinkova-Kostova, Albena T., et al. "KEAP1 and Done? Targeting the NRF2 Pathway with Sulforaphane." *Trends in Food Science & Technology*, vol. 69, no. Pt B, Nov. 2017, pp. 257–69. *PubMed Central*, doi:10.1016/j.tifs.2017.02.002.

35. Martínez-Huélamo, Miriam, et al. "Modulation of Nrf2 by Olive Oil and Wine Polyphenols and Neuroprotection." *Antioxidants*, vol. 6, no. 4, Sept. 2017. *PubMed Central*, doi:10.3390/antiox6040073.

Chapter 5: Getting Rid of the Toxicants that Decrease the Quality of Your Eggs

1. Patel, Shreya, et al. "Effects of Endocrine-Disrupting Chemicals on the Ovary." *Biology of Reproduction*, vol. 93, no. 1, July 2015.

2. Horan, Tegan S., et al. "Replacement Bisphenols Adversely Affect Mouse Gametogenesis with Consequences for Subsequent Generations." *Current Biology: CB*, vol. 28, no. 18, 24 2018, pp. 2948-2954.e3.

3. Chun, Yang Z., et al. "Most Plastic Products Release Estrogenic Chemicals: A Potential Health Problem That Can Be Solved." *Environmental Health Perspectives*, vol. 119, no. 7, July 2011, pp. 989–96.

4. Wang, Wei, et al. "In Utero Bisphenol A Exposure Disrupts Germ Cell Nest Breakdown and Reduces Fertility with Age in the Mouse." *Toxicology and Applied Pharmacology*, vol. 276, no. 2, Apr. 2014, pp. 157–64.

5. Yuan, Mu, et al. "Environmentally Relevant Levels of Bisphenol A Affect Uterine Decidualization and Embryo Implantation through the Estrogen Receptor/Serum and Glucocorticoid-Regulated Kinase 1/Epithelial Sodium Ion Channel α-Subunit Pathway in a Mouse Model." *Fertility and Sterility*, vol. 109, no. 4, 2018, pp. 735-744.e1.

6. Hunt, Patricia A., et al. "Bisphenol a Exposure Causes Meiotic Aneuploidy in the Female Mouse." *Current Biology: CB*, vol. 13, no. 7, Apr. 2003, pp. 546–53.

7. Tomza-Marciniak, Agnieszka, et al. "Effect of Bisphenol A on Reproductive Processes: A Review of in Vitro, in Vivo and Epidemiological Studies." *Journal of Applied Toxicology: JAT*, vol. 38, no. 1, Jan. 2018, pp. 51–80.

8. Mok-Lin, E., et al. "Urinary Bisphenol A Concentrations and Ovarian Response among Women Undergoing IVF." *International Journal of Andrology*, vol. 33, no. 2, Apr. 2010, pp. 385–93.

9. Ziv-Gal, Ayelet, and Jodi A. Flaws. "Evidence for Bisphenol A-Induced Female Infertility - Review (2007–2016)." *Fertility and Sterility*, vol. 106, no. 4, Sept. 2016, pp. 827–56.

10. Zhang, Mianqun, et al. "Melatonin Protects Oocyte Quality from Bisphenol A-Induced Deterioration in the Mouse." *Journal of Pineal Research*, vol. 62, no. 3, Apr. 2017.

11. Liao, Chunyang, and Kurunthachalam Kannan. "Concentrations and Profiles of Bisphenol A and Other Bisphenol Analogues in Foodstuffs from the United States and Their Implications for Human Exposure." *Journal of Agricultural and Food Chemistry*, vol. 61, no. 19, May 2013, pp. 4655–62.

12. Lorber, Matthew, et al. "Exposure Assessment of Adult Intake of Bisphenol A (BPA) with Emphasis on Canned Food Dietary Exposures." *Environment International*, vol. 77, Apr. 2015, pp. 55–62.

13. LaKind, Judy S., and Daniel Q. Naiman. "Daily Intake of Bisphenol A and Potential Sources of Exposure: 2005–2006 National Health and Nutrition Examination Survey." *Journal of Exposure Science & Environmental Epidemiology*, vol. 21, no. 3, May 2011, pp. 272–79.

14. Hauser, Russ, et al. "Urinary Phthalate Metabolite Concentrations and Reproductive Outcomes among Women Undergoing in Vitro Fertilization: Results from the

EARTH Study." *Environmental Health Perspectives*, vol. 124, no. 6, 2016, pp. 831–39.

15. Machtinger, Ronit, et al. "Urinary Concentrations of Biomarkers of Phthalates and Phthalate Alternatives and IVF Outcomes." *Environment International*, vol. 111, Feb. 2018, pp. 23–31.

16. Xu, Ren-ai, et al. "Structure-Activity Relationships of Phthalates in Inhibition of Human Placental 3β-Hydroxysteroid Dehydrogenase 1 and Aromatase." *Reproductive Toxicology*, vol. 61, June 2016, pp. 151–61.

17. Sen, Nivedita, et al. "Short Term Exposure to Di-n-Butyl Phthalate (DBP) Disrupts Ovarian Function in Young CD-1 Mice." *Reproductive Toxicology*, vol. 53, June 2015, pp. 15–22.

18. Al-Saleh, Iman, et al. "Couples Exposure to Phthalates and Its Influence on in Vitro Fertilization Outcomes." *Chemosphere*, vol. 226, July 2019, pp. 597–606.

19. Messerlian, Carmen, et al. "Urinary Concentrations of Phthalate Metabolites and Pregnancy Loss Among Women Conceiving with Medically Assisted Reproduction." Epidemiology, vol. 27, no. 6, Nov. 2016, p. 879.

20. Koniecki, Diane, et al. "Phthalates in Cosmetic and Personal Care Products: Concentrations and Possible Dermal Exposure." *Environmental Research*, vol. 111, no. 3, Apr. 2011, pp. 329–36.

21. Philips, Elise M., et al. "First Trimester Urinary Bisphenol and Phthalate Concentrations and Time to Pregnancy: A Population-Based Cohort Analysis." *The Journal of Clinical Endocrinology and Metabolism*, vol. 103, no. 9, 01 2018, pp. 3540–47.

Chapter 6: Improving Mitochondrial Function in Your Eggs

1. St John, Justin C., et al. "Mitochondrial DNA Supplementation as an Enhancer of Female Reproductive

Capacity." *Current Opinion in Obstetrics & Gynecology*, vol. 28, no. 3, 2016, pp. 211–16.

2. Schutt, Amy K., et al. "Preovulatory Exposure to a Protein-Restricted Diet Disrupts Amino Acid Kinetics and Alters Mitochondrial Structure and Function in the Rat Oocyte and Is Partially Rescued by Folic Acid."*Reproductive Biology and Endocrinology : RB&E*, vol. 17, Jan. 2019.

3. Ou, Xiang-Hong, et al. "Maternal Insulin Resistance Causes Oxidative Stress and Mitochondrial Dysfunction in Mouse Oocytes." *Human Reproduction (Oxford, England)*, vol. 27, no. 7, July 2012, pp. 2130–45.

4. Madreiter-Sokolowski, Corina T., et al. "Targeting Mitochondria to Counteract Age-Related Cellular Dysfunction." *Genes*, vol. 9, no. 3, Mar. 2018.

5. Ben-Meir, Assaf, et al. "Coenzyme Q10 Restores Oocyte Mitochondrial Function and Fertility during Reproductive Aging." *Aging Cell*, vol. 14, no. 5, Oct. 2015, pp. 887–95.

6. Yamanaka, Ryu, et al. "Mitochondrial Mg2+ Homeostasis Decides Cellular Energy Metabolism and Vulnerability to Stress." *Scientific Reports*, vol. 6, July 2016. *PubMed Central*, doi:10.1038/srep30027.

Chapter 7: Sleep and Melatonin: A Key to Conception

1. Rocha, R. M. P., et al. "Interaction between Melatonin and Follicle-Stimulating Hormone Promotes in Vitro Development of Caprine Preantral Follicles." *Domestic Animal Endocrinology*, vol. 44, no. 1, Jan. 2013, pp. 1–9.

2. Tagliaferri, Valeria, et al. "Melatonin Treatment May Be Able to Restore Menstrual Cyclicity in Women With PCOS: A Pilot Study." *Reproductive Sciences (Thousand Oaks, Calif.)*, vol. 25, no. 2, Feb. 2018, pp. 269–75.

3. Tamura, Hiroshi, et al. "The Role of Melatonin as an Antioxidant in the Follicle." *Journal of Ovarian Research*, vol. 5, Jan. 2012, p. 5.

4. Pacchiarotti, Alessandro, et al. "Effect of Myo-Inositol and Melatonin versus Myo-Inositol, in a Randomized Controlled Trial, for Improving in Vitro Fertilization of Patients with Polycystic Ovarian Syndrome." *Gynecological Endocrinology: The Official Journal of the International Society of Gynecological Endocrinology* , vol. 32, no. 1, 2016, pp. 69–73.

Chapter 8: What Should You Eat to Enhance Your Odds of Getting Pregnant?

1. Vujkovic, Marijana, et al. "The Preconception Mediterranean Dietary Pattern in Couples Undergoing in Vitro Fertilization/Intracytoplasmic Sperm Injection Treatment Increases the Chance of Pregnancy." *Fertility and Sterility*, vol. 94, no. 6, Nov. 2010, pp. 2096–101.

2. Jahangirifar, Maryam, et al. "Dietary Patterns and The Outcomes of Assisted Reproductive Techniques in Women with Primary Infertility: A Prospective Cohort Study." *International Journal of Fertility & Sterility*, vol. 12, no. 4, Jan. 2019, pp. 316–23.

3. Snow, R. C., et al. "High Dietary Fiber and Low Saturated Fat Intake among Oligomenorrheic Undergraduates." *Fertility and Sterility*, vol. 54, no. 4, Oct. 1990, pp. 632–37.

4. Dunneram, Yashvee, et al. "Dietary Intake and Age at Natural Menopause: Results from the UK Women's Cohort Study." *Journal of Epidemiology and Community Health*, vol. 72, no. 8, 2018, pp. 733–40.

5. Baines, Surinder, et al. "How Does the Health and Well-Being of Young Australian Vegetarian and Semi-Vegetarian Women Compare with Non-Vegetarians?" *Public Health Nutrition*, vol. 10, no. 5, May 2007, pp. 436–42.

6. Singh, Meharban. "Essential Fatty Acids, DHA and Human Brain." *Indian Journal of Pediatrics*, vol. 72, no. 3, Mar. 2005, pp. 239–42.

7. Zhang, Zhiying, et al. "Dietary Intakes of EPA and DHA Omega-3 Fatty Acids among US Childbearing-Age and Pregnant Women: An Analysis of NHANES 2001–2014." *Nutrients*, vol. 10, no. 4, Mar. 2018.

8. Nehra, Deepika, et al. "Prolonging the Female Reproductive Lifespan and Improving Egg Quality with Dietary Omega-3 Fatty Acids." *Aging Cell*, vol. 11, no. 6, Dec. 2012, pp. 1046–54.

9. Gaskins, Audrey J., et al. "Seafood Intake, Sexual Activity, and Time to Pregnancy." *The Journal of Clinical Endocrinology & Metabolism*, vol. 103, no. 7, July 2018, pp. 2680–88.

10. Safarinejad, M. R. "Effect of Omega-3 Polyunsaturated Fatty Acid Supplementation on Semen Profile and Enzymatic Anti-Oxidant Capacity of Seminal Plasma in Infertile Men with Idiopathic Oligoasthenoteratospermia: A Double-Blind, Placebo-Controlled, Randomised Study." *Andrologia*, vol. 43, no. 1, Feb. 2011, pp. 38–47.

11. Chiu, Y. H., et al. "Serum Omega-3 Fatty Acids and Treatment Outcomes among Women Undergoing Assisted Reproduction." *Human Reproduction (Oxford, England)*, vol. 33, no. 1, Jan. 2018, pp. 156–65.

12. Olsen, S. F., et al. "Plasma Concentrations of Long Chain N-3 Fatty Acids in Early and Mid-Pregnancy and Risk of Early Preterm Birth." *EBioMedicine*, vol. 35, Aug. 2018, pp. 325–33.

13. Carlson, Susan E., et al. "DHA Supplementation and Pregnancy Outcomes123." *The American Journal of Clinical Nutrition*, vol. 97, no. 4, Apr. 2013, pp. 808–15.

14. Braarud, Hanne Cecilie, et al. "Maternal DHA Status during Pregnancy Has a Positive Impact on Infant Problem Solving: A Norwegian Prospective Observation Study." *Nutrients*, vol. 10, no. 5, Apr. 2018.

15. Nutrition, Center for Food Safety and Applied. "FDA/EPA 2004 Advice on What You Need to Know About Mercury in Fish and Shellfish." *FDA*, July 2019.

16. EWG's Consumer Guide to Seafood." EWG, https://www.ewg.org/research/ewgs-good-seafood-guide.

17. Taha, Ameer Y., et al. "Dietary Omega-6 Fatty Acid Lowering Increases Bioavailability of Omega-3 Polyunsaturated Fatty Acids in Human Plasma Lipid Pools." *Prostaglandins, Leukotrienes, and Essential Fatty Acids*, vol. 90, no. 5, May 2014, pp. 151–57.

18. Kazemi, Ashraf, et al. "Does Dietary Fat Intake Influence Oocyte Competence and Embryo Quality by Inducing Oxidative Stress in Follicular Fluid?" *Iranian Journal of Reproductive Medicine*, vol. 11, no. 12, Dec. 2013, pp. 1005–12.

19. Russell, J. B., et al. "Does Changing a Patient's Dietary Consumption of Proteins and Carbohydrates Impact Blastocyst Development and Clinical Pregnancy Rates from One Cycle to the Next?" *Fertility and Sterility* , vol. 98, no. 3, Sept. 2012, p. S47.

20. Chiu, Yu-Han, et al. "Association Between Pesticide Residue Intake From Consumption of Fruits and Vegetables and Pregnancy Outcomes Among Women Undergoing Infertility Treatment With Assisted Reproductive Technology." JAMA *Internal Medicine*, vol. 178, no. 1, Jan. 2018, pp. 17–26.

21. Chiu, Y. H., et al. "Fruit and Vegetable Intake and Their Pesticide Residues in Relation to Semen Quality among Men from a Fertility Clinic." *Human Reproduction*, vol. 30, no. 6, June 2015, pp. 1342–51.

22. Chiu, Yu-Han, et al. "Intake of Fruits and Vegetables with Low-to-Moderate Pesticide Residues Is Positively Associated with Semen-Quality Parameters among Young Healthy Men." *The Journal of Nutrition*, vol. 146, no. 5, May 2016, pp. 1084–92.

Chapter 9: Leptin: A Hormone that Links Your Weight to Fertility

1. van der Steeg, Jan Willem, et al. "Obesity Affects Spontaneous Pregnancy Chances in Subfertile, Ovulatory Women." *Human Reproduction (Oxford, England)*, vol. 23, no. 2, Feb. 2008, pp. 324–28.

2. Rich-Edwards, Janet W., et al. "Physical Activity, Body Mass Index, and Ovulatory Disorder Infertility." *Epidemiology*, vol. 13, no. 2, Mar. 2002, p. 184.

3. Cai, Jiali, et al. "Low Body Mass Index Compromises Live Birth Rate in Fresh Transfer in Vitro Fertilization Cycles: A Retrospective Study in a Chinese Population." *Fertility and Sterility*, vol. 107, no. 2, 2017, pp. 422-429.e2.

4. Pérez-Pérez, Antonio, et al. "Leptin Action in Normal and Pathological Pregnancies." *Journal of Cellular and Molecular Medicine*, vol. 22, no. 2, Feb. 2018, pp. 716–27.

5. Reference, Genetics Home. "Congenital Leptin Deficiency." *Genetics Home Reference*, https://ghr.nlm.nih.gov/condition/congenital-leptin-deficiency.

6. Odle, Angela K., et al. "Leptin Regulation of Gonadotrope Gonadotropin-Releasing Hormone Receptors As a Metabolic Checkpoint and Gateway to Reproductive Competence." *Frontiers in Endocrinology*, vol. 8, Jan. 2018.

7. Chou, Sharon H., et al. "Leptin Is an Effective Treatment for Hypothalamic Amenorrhea." *Proceedings of the National Academy of Sciences*, vol. 108, no. 16, Apr. 2011, pp. 6585–90.

8. Torstveit, M. K., and J. Sundgot-Borgen. "Participation in Leanness Sports but Not Training Volume Is Associated with Menstrual Dysfunction: A National Survey of 1276 Elite Athletes and Controls." *British Journal of Sports Medicine*, vol. 39, no. 3, Mar. 2005, pp. 141–47.

9. Kamyabi, Zahra, and Tayebe Gholamalizade. "A Comparative Study of Serum and Follicular Fluid Leptin

among Explained Infertile, Unexplained and Fertile Women." *International Journal of Fertility & Sterility*, vol. 9, no. 2, 2015, pp. 150–56.

10. Lv, Dongying, et al. "Leptin Mediates the Effects of Melatonin on Female Reproduction in Mammals." *Journal of Pineal Research*, vol. 66, no. 3, Apr. 2019, p. e12559.

11. Figueiro, Mariana, et al. "Light Modulates Leptin and Ghrelin in Sleep-Restricted Adults." International Journal of Endocrinology, Volume 2012, Article ID 530726

Chapter 10: Lifestyle Changes that Promote Fertility

1. Foucaut, Aude-Marie, et al. "Sedentary Behavior, Physical Inactivity and Body Composition in Relation to Idiopathic Infertility among Men and Women." *PloS One*, vol. 14, no. 4, 2019, p. e0210770.

2. Cialdella-Kam, Lynn, et al. "Dietary Intervention Restored Menses in Female Athletes with Exercise-Associated Menstrual Dysfunction with Limited Impact on Bone and Muscle Health." *Nutrients*, vol. 6, no. 8, July 2014, pp. 3018–39.

3. Wise, Lauren A., et al. "A Prospective Cohort Study of Physical Activity and Time to Pregnancy." *Fertility and Sterility*, vol. 97, no. 5, May 2012, pp. 1136-1142.e1-4.

4. Cialdella-Kam, Lynn, et al. "Vegetarian, Gluten-Free, and Energy Restricted Diets in Female Athletes." *Sports*, vol. 4, no. 4, Oct. 2016.

5. Mitro, Susanna D., et al. "Consumer Chemicals in Indoor Dust: A Quantitative-Analysis of U.S. Studies." *Environmental Science & Technology*, vol. 50, no. 19, Oct. 2016, pp. 10661–72.

6. Saini, Amandeep, et al. "From Clothing to Laundry Water: Investigating the Fate of Phthalates, Brominated Flame Retardants, and Organophosphate Esters." *Environmental Science & Technology*, vol. 50, no. 17, 06 2016, pp. 9289–97.

7. Nepomnaschy, Pablo A., et al. "Cortisol Levels and Very Early Pregnancy Loss in Humans." *Proceedings of the National Academy of Sciences of the United States of America* , vol. 103, no. 10, Mar. 2006, pp. 3938–42.

8. Guyon, Aurore, et al. "Effects of Insufficient Sleep on Pituitary–Adrenocortical Response to CRH Stimulation in Healthy Men." *Sleep*, vol. 40, no. 6, Apr. 2017.

9. Sullivan, Molly, et al. "The Effects of Power and Stretch Yoga on Affect and Salivary Cortisol in Women." *Journal of Health Psychology*, vol. 24, no. 12, Oct. 2019, pp. 1658–67.

10. Turakitwanakan, Wanpen, et al. "Effects of Mindfulness Meditation on Serum Cortisol of Medical Students." *Journal of the Medical Association of Thailand = Chotmaihet Thangphaet* , vol. 96 Suppl 1, Jan. 2013, pp. S90-95.

11. Azuma, Kagaku, et al. "Association between Mastication, the Hippocampus, and the HPA Axis: A Comprehensive Review." *International Journal of Molecular Sciences*, vol. 18, no. 8, Aug. 2017.

12. Park, Bum Jin, et al. "The Physiological Effects of Shinrin-Yoku (Taking in the Forest Atmosphere or Forest Bathing): Evidence from Field Experiments in 24 Forests across Japan." *Environmental Health and Preventive Medicine*, vol. 15, no. 1, Jan. 2010, pp. 18–26.

13. Chandrasekhar, K., et al. "A Prospective, Randomized Double-Blind, Placebo-Controlled Study of Safety and Efficacy of a High-Concentration Full-Spectrum Extract of Ashwagandha Root in Reducing Stress and Anxiety in Adults." *Indian Journal of Psychological Medicine*, vol. 34, no. 3, July 2012, pp. 255–62.

14. Jothie Richard, Edwin, et al. "Anti-Stress Activity of Ocimum Sanctum: Possible Effects on Hypothalamic-Pituitary-Adrenal Axis." *Phytotherapy Research: PTR*, vol. 30, no. 5, May 2016, pp. 805–14.

Chapter 11: Supplements for Enhancing Fertility

1. Mohn, Emily S., et al. "Evidence of Drug–Nutrient Interactions with Chronic Use of Commonly Prescribed Medications: An Update." *Pharmaceutics*, vol. 10, no. 1, Mar. 2018.

2. Pawlak, Roman, et al. "How Prevalent Is Vitamin B(12) Deficiency among Vegetarians?" *Nutrition Reviews*, vol. 71, no. 2, Feb. 2013, pp. 110–17.

3. Paffoni, Alessio, et al. "Homocysteine Pathway and in Vitro Fertilization Outcome." Reproductive Toxicology (Elmsford, N.Y.), vol. 76, 2018, pp. 12–16.

4. La Vecchia, Irene, et al. "Folate, Homocysteine and Selected Vitamins and Minerals Status in Infertile Women." *The European Journal of Contraception & Reproductive Health Care: The Official Journal of the European Society of Contraception* , vol. 22, no. 1, Feb. 2017, pp. 70–75.

5. Boxmeer, Jolanda C., et al. "IVF Outcomes Are Associated with Biomarkers of the Homocysteine Pathway in Monofollicular Fluid." *Human Reproduction (Oxford, England)*, vol. 24, no. 5, May 2009, pp. 1059–66.

6. Boxmeer, Jolanda C., et al. "Seminal Plasma Cobalamin Significantly Correlates with Sperm Concentration in Men Undergoing IVF or ICSI Procedures." *Journal of Andrology*, vol. 28, no. 4, Aug. 2007, pp. 521–27.

7. Huijgen, Nicole A., et al. "Effect of Medications for Gastric Acid-Related Symptoms on Total Motile Sperm Count and Concentration: A Case–Control Study in Men of Subfertile Couples from the Netherlands." *Drug Safety*, vol. 40, no. 3, 2017, pp. 241–48.

8. Raghavan, Ramkripa, et al. "Maternal Multivitamin Intake, Plasma Folate and Vitamin B12 Levels and Autism Spectrum Disorder Risk in Offspring." Paediatric and Perinatal Epidemiology, vol. 32, no. 1, 2018, pp. 100–11.

9. Wiens, Darrell, and M. Catherine DeSoto. "Is High Folic Acid Intake a Risk Factor for Autism?–A Review." *Brain Sciences*, vol. 7, no. 11, Nov. 2017.

10. Patanwala, Imran, et al. "Folic Acid Handling by the Human Gut: Implications for Food Fortification and Supplementation." *The American Journal of Clinical Nutrition*, vol. 100, no. 2, Aug. 2014, pp. 593–99.

11. Nymark, Ole, et al. "Nutritional 1C Imbalance, B12 Tissue Accumulation, and Pregnancy Outcomes: An Experimental Study in Rats." *Nutrients*, vol. 10, no. 11, Oct. 2018.

12. Rudick, Briana J., et al. "Influence of Vitamin D Levels on in Vitro Fertilization Outcomes in Donor-Recipient Cycles."*Fertility and Sterility*, vol. 101, no. 2, Feb. 2014, pp. 447–52. *www.fertstert.org*, doi:10.1016/j.fertstert.2013.10.008.

13. Dabrowski, Filip A., et al. "The Role of Vitamin D in Reproductive Health–A Trojan Horse or the Golden Fleece?" *Nutrients*, vol. 7, no. 6, May 2015, pp. 4139–53.

14. Heaney, Robert P., et al. "Vitamin D3 Is More Potent Than Vitamin D2 in Humans." *The Journal of Clinical Endocrinology & Metabolism*, vol. 96, no. 3, Mar. 2011, pp. E447–52.

15. Liu, Yifan, et al. "Age-Related Changes in the Mitochondria of Human Mural Granulosa Cells." *Human Reproduction (Oxford, England)*, vol. 32, no. 12, Dec. 2017, pp. 2465–73.

16. Ben-Meir, Assaf, et al. "Coenzyme Q10 Restores Oocyte Mitochondrial Function and Fertility during Reproductive Aging." *Aging Cell*, vol. 14, no. 5, Oct. 2015, pp. 887–95.

17. Xu, Yangying, et al. "Pretreatment with Coenzyme Q10 Improves Ovarian Response and Embryo Quality in Low-Prognosis Young Women with Decreased Ovarian Reserve: A Randomized Controlled Trial." *Reproductive Biology and Endocrinology: RB&E*, vol. 16, no. 1, Mar. 2018, p. 29.

18. Safarinejad, Mohammad Reza, et al. "Effects of the Reduced Form of Coenzyme Q10 (Ubiquinol) on Semen Parameters in Men with Idiopathic Infertility: A Double-Blind, Placebo Controlled, Randomized Study." *The Journal of Urology*, vol. 188, no. 2, Aug. 2012, pp. 526–31.

19. Ben-Meir, Assaf, et al. "Coenzyme Q10 Restores Oocyte Mitochondrial Function and Fertility during Reproductive Aging." *Aging Cell*, vol. 14, no. 5, Oct. 2015, pp. 887–95.

20. Naredi, Nikita, et al. "Dehydroepiandrosterone: A Panacea for the Ageing Ovary?" *Medical Journal, Armed Forces India*, vol. 71, no. 3, July 2015, pp. 274–77.

21. Schwarze, Juan Enrique, et al. "DHEA Use to Improve Likelihood of IVF/ICSI Success in Patients with Diminished Ovarian Reserve: A Systematic Review and Meta-Analysis." *JBRA Assisted Reproduction*, vol. 22, no. 4, Nov. 2018, pp. 369–74.

22. Hu, Qiaofei, et al. "The Effect of Dehydroepiandrosterone Supplementation on Ovarian Response Is Associated with Androgen Receptor in Diminished Ovarian Reserve Women." *Journal of Ovarian Research*, vol. 10, no. 1, May 2017, p. 32.

23. Gleicher, Norbert, et al. "The Importance of Adrenal Hypoandrogenism in Infertile Women with Low Functional Ovarian Reserve: A Case Study of Associated Adrenal Insufficiency." *Reproductive Biology and Endocrinology: RB&E*, vol. 14, Apr. 2016. *PubMed Central*, doi:10.1186/s12958-016-0158-9.

24. Lennartsson, Anna-Karin, et al. "Perceived Stress at Work Is Associated with Lower Levels of DHEA-S." *PLoS ONE*, vol. 8, no. 8, Aug. 2013.

25. Lai, Hung-Min, et al. "Higher DHEAS Levels Associated with Long-Term Practicing of Tai Chi." *The Chinese Journal of Physiology*, vol. 60, no. 2, Apr. 2017, pp. 124–30. *PubMed*, doi:10.4077/CJP.2017.BAF454.

Chapter 12: Testing Your Nutritional Status

1. Ozkan, Sebiha, et al. "Replete Vitamin D Stores Predict Reproductive Success Following IVF." *Fertility and Sterility*, vol. 94, no. 4, Sept. 2010, pp. 1314–19.

2. Hollis, Bruce W., and Carol L. Wagner. "New Insights into the Vitamin D Requirements during Pregnancy." *Bone Research*, vol. 5, 2017, p. 17030.

3. Kawai, Tomoko, et al. "De Novo-Synthesized Retinoic Acid in Ovarian Antral Follicles Enhances FSH-Mediated Ovarian Follicular Cell Differentiation and Female Fertility." *Endocrinology*, vol. 157, no. 5, May 2016, pp. 2160–72.

4. Thaler, Christian J., et al. "Effects of the Common 677C>T Mutation of the 5,10-Methylenetetrahydrofolate Reductase (MTHFR) Gene on Ovarian Responsiveness to Recombinant Follicle-Stimulating Hormone."*American Journal of Reproductive Immunology*, vol. 55, no. 4, 2006, pp. 251–58.

5. Pacchiarotti, Arianna, et al. "The Possible Role of Hyperhomocysteinemia on IVF Outcome." *Journal of Assisted Reproduction and Genetics*, vol. 24, no. 10, Oct. 2007, pp. 459–62.

6. Škovierová, Henrieta, et al. "The Molecular and Cellular Effect of Homocysteine Metabolism Imbalance on Human Health." *International Journal of Molecular Sciences*, vol. 17, no. 10, Oct. 2016. *PubMed Central*, doi:10.3390/ijms17101733.

7. Verma, Indu, et al. "Prevalence of Hypothyroidism in Infertile Women and Evaluation of Response of Treatment for Hypothyroidism on Infertility." *International Journal of Applied and Basic Medical Research*, vol. 2, no. 1, 2012, pp. 17–19.

Chapter 13: What About Your Partner?

1. Geoffroy-Siraudin, Cendrine, et al. "Decline of Semen Quality among 10 932 Males Consulting for Couple Infertility over a 20-Year Period in Marseille, France." *Asian Journal of Andrology*, vol. 14, no. 4, July 2012, pp. 584–90.

2. Centola, G. M., et al. "Decline in Sperm Count and Motility in Young Adult Men from 2003 to 2013: Observations from a U.S. Sperm Bank." *Andrology*, vol. 4, no. 2, Mar. 2016, pp. 270–76.

3. Bloom, M. S., et al. "Associations between Urinary Phthalate Concentrations and Semen Quality Parameters in a General Population." *Human Reproduction (Oxford, England)*, vol. 30, no. 11, Nov. 2015, pp. 2645–57.

4. Broe, A., et al. "Association between Use of Phthalate-Containing Medication and Semen Quality among Men in Couples Referred for Assisted Reproduction." *Human Reproduction (Oxford, England)*, vol. 33, no. 3, Mar. 2018, pp. 503–11.

5. Guo, Ying, et al. "Melatonin Ameliorates Restraint Stress-Induced Oxidative Stress and Apoptosis in Testicular Cells via NF-KB/INOS and Nrf2/ HO-1 Signaling Pathway." *Scientific Reports*, vol. 7, Aug. 2017.

6. Salas-Huetos, Albert, et al. "Dietary Patterns, Foods and Nutrients in Male Fertility Parameters and Fecundability: A Systematic Review of Observational Studies." *Human Reproduction Update*, vol. 23, no. 4, July 2017, pp. 371–89.

.

Acknowledgments

This book has been 20 years in the making...ever since I first opened my clinic doors to patients.

I owe the beginning of my trip down the fertility rabbit hole to my very first fertility patient, Martha C. Ever since then I knew this is where I belong.

To every single one of my clients, thank you for allowing me to share your journey. I learn so much from each and every one of you.

Many, many thanks to...

Debbie Moon, without you, this would not have been possible.

My clients who read the manuscript and provided valuable feedback. That's you, K.B., A.E., L.T., M.B.

Dr. Arlene Morales for your comments and support throughout the years.

Anamitra Roy - your resourcefulness and dedication allows me to focus on what's important.

Bonnie DeGraw - your inner light shines so bright that there is no choice but to be swept up in your loving embrace.

Chia Chia Cheng - a kinder, more compassionate person one would be hardpressed to find. Your incisive discernment of any situation never ceases to amaze me.

East Phillips - you awe me with your creativity. Let me catch my breath as I try to keep up with you.

Ma and Ba – I would not be here without you. Literally.

Davy Chang – strong, steadfast, intrepid...a superhero in every regards.

And, of course, my kids...the joy I've experienced with you both fuels my purpose to help other women become mothers as well. Jia you.

.

About the Author

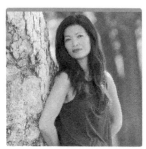 Julie Chang is a licensed acupuncturist with a clinical practice specializing in helping women in their 30s and 40s get pregnant.

She has been in practice since 2000. Over the years, as more women from all over the world reached out for help, she expanded her services to offer online fertility coaching to help women overcome fertility issues. She can be found at *www.FertilityEggspurt.com*.

With a Bachelor of Science in Microbiology and Molecular Genetics and Master in Traditional Oriental Medicine (Magna Cum Laude), she blends natural approaches tested by time with modern strategies backed by science.

Teaching others to heal their bodies safely and naturally is Ms. Chang's passion and life. She practices the same health principles she advises her clients, so she has personally experienced the power of healing from within.

Ms. Chang spends her free time with her children, friends, and family. She loves trying new restaurants and finding new experiences wherever she is – at home or when traveling. She enjoys yoga, hip hop class, and getting her reps in at the gym. Her constant companion is her fur baby, Oreo.

Printed in Poland
by Amazon Fulfillment
Poland Sp. z o.o., Wrocław

80349227R00110